TEXTBOOK FOR BHMS STUDENTS

Pioneers of Homoeopathy

ILLUSTRATED BIOGRAPHIES OF PERSONALITIES & THEIR CONTRIBUTIONS

B. JAIN PUBLISHERS PVT. LTD.

PIONEERS OF HOMOEOPATHY
ILLUSTRATED BIOGRAPHIES OF PERSONALITIES & THEIR CONTRIBUTIONS

***First Edition* : 2003**

Price Rs. 175.00

Published by Kuldeep Jain for
B. Jain Publishers (P) Ltd.
1921, Street No. 10, Chuna Mandi,
Paharganj, New Delhi 110 055 (INDIA)
Phones: 2358 0800, 51698991,
2358 3100, 2358 1300, 2358 1100,
Fax: 2358 0471, 51698993
Email: bjain@vsnl.com
***Website:* www.bjainbooks.com**

Printed in India by
J.J. Offset Printers
522, FIE, Patpar Ganj, Delhi - 110 092

ISBN: 81-8056-387-1 **BOOK CODE : BB-5732**

PUBLISHER'S NOTES

This book is about the lives of founder and early leaders of homoeopathy. We have read their invaluable literature, we have seen their treatment of incurable diseases. But in this book we read about their circumstances, their family, their students, their teachers, this followers, their contributions, their professional successes and challenges.

Material for this book has come from numerous sources and it was a task compiling and editing it. We are thankful to Dr. Mahendra Singh who has contributed about 50% of the material.

We also thank the many learned advisors and contributors who all along gave great support to the production of this book.

We faced a lot of difficulties while working on this book – the life history of many important homoeopaths is not available, many photographs are not available, especially of Indian homoeopaths.

In view of the above, readers are requested to send us any information to include more *Pioneers* in future editions of this book. This kind of book is only possible through a combined effort of all of us. We will acknowledge your name for any material which is supplied by you.

The book has been specially designed for Ist year BHMS students according to CCH syllabus.

Dr. P.N. Jain

THIS BOOK IS DEDICATED TO THE MEMORY OF ALL THE GREAT HOMOEOPATHS MENTIONED AND NOT MENTIONED WITHIN THIS BOOK

CONTENTS

SECTION-A (7 to 9)

A-1 Dr. Allen, Henry C. (Born: 02-10-1830 / Died: 22-01-1909) 8
A-2 Dr. Allen, Timothy Field (Born: 24-04-1837 / Died: 05-12-1902) 9

SECTION-B (11 to 46)

B-1 Dr. Banerjee, R.M. (Born: 28-11-1919 / Died: 09-04-1977) 12
B-2 Dr. Banerjee, Sripada (Died: 1966) 13
B-3 Dr. Bhatia, Anil (Born: 13-05-1942 / Died: 12-10-2002) 14
B-4 Dr. Boenninghausen, Clemens Maria Franz Von (Born: 12-03-1785 / Died: 26-01-1864) 17
B-5 Dr. Boericke, William (Born: 26-11-1849 / Died: 01-04-1929) 26
B-6 Dr. Boger, Cyrus Maxwell (Born: 13-05-1861 / Died: 02-09-1935) 28
B-7 Dr. Bose, B.K. (Born: 1879 / Died: 16-12-1977) 30
B-8 Dr. Burnett, James Compton (Born: 10-07-1840 / Died: 02-04-1901) 37
B-9 Dr. Byod, William Earnest (Born: 21-05-1891 / Died: 1955) 44
B-10 Dr. Bysack, Hem Chandra (Born: 1963) 46

SECTION-C (47 to 65)

C-1 Dr. Caspari, Carl (Born: 1798 / Died: 15-02-1828) 48
C-2 Dr. Chand, Diwan (Born: 03-08-1887 / Died: 14-05-1961) 52
C-3 Dr. Chatterjee, D. N. (Born: 1903 / Died: 1961) 59
C-4 Dr. Chowdhury, Bankim (Born: 1904 / Died: 1977) 60
C-5 Dr. Clarke, John Henry (Born: 1853 / Died: 24-11-1931) 62
C-6 Dr. Close, Stuart M. (Born: 14-11-1860 / Died: 26-05-1929) 65

SECTION-D (67 to 94)

D-1 Dr. Daftari, K.L. (Born: 22-11-1880 / Died: 19-02-1956) 68
D-2 Dr. Das, Rai Bahadur Bishambar (Born: 21-03-1891 / Died: 12-07-1965) .69
D-3 Dr. De, D.N. (Born: 1877 / Died: 19-09-1943) 70
D-4 Dr. Dev, Khan Chand (Died: 1941) 71
D-5 Dr. Desai, Maganlal B. (Born: 1906 / Died: 1977) 72
D-6 Dr. Dewey, Willis A. (Born: 25-10-1858 / Died: 01-04-1938) 74
D-7 Dr. Dhawale, Laxman Dinchura (Born: 21-07-1884 / Died: 10-12-1960)..75
D-8 Dr. Dudgeon, Robert Ellis (Born: 17-03-1829 / Died: 18-09-1904) 76
D-9 Dr. Dunham, Carroll (Born: 29-10-1828 / Died: 18-02-1877) 83
D-10 Dr. Dutt, Rajendra Lall (Born: 1818 / Died: 05-06-1889) 94

SECTION-F (95 to 102)

D-1 Dr. Farrington, Ernest A. (Born: 01-01-1847 / Died: 15-12-1885) 96
D-2 Dr. Franz, Karl Gottlab (Born: 08-05-1795 / Died: 08-11-1835) 100

SECTION-G (103 to 127)

G-1 Dr. Ghatak, Nilmani (Born: 1872 / Died: 19-01-1940) 104
G-2 Dr. Ghosh, S.C. (Born: 1870 / Died: 1953) 107
G-3 Dr. Gross, Gustav Wilhelm (Born: 06-09-1794 / Died: 18-09-1847) 118
G-4 Dr. Guernsey, Henry Newell (Born: 10-02-1817 / Died: 27-06-1885) 125
G-5 Dr. Gururaju, M. (Born: 1897 / Died: 25-11-1963) 126

SECTION-H (129 to 166)

H-1 Dr. Hahnemann, Christian Friedrich Samuel (Born: 10-04-1755 / Died: 02-07-1843) 130
H-2 Dr. Hahnemann, Melanie d'Hervilly Gohier (Born: 02-02-1800 / Died: 27-05-1878) 139

H-3 Dr. Hartmann, Franz (Born: 18-05-1796 / Died: 10-10-1853) 141
H-4 Dr. Hazra, J. N. 145
H-5 Dr. Hempel, Charles Julius (Born: 05-09-1811 / Died: 24-09-1879) 146
H-6 Dr. Hering, Constantine (Born: 01-01-1800 / Died: 23-07-1880) 157
H-7 Dr. Honigberger, John Martin 161
H-8 Dr. Hughes, Richard (Born: 1836 / Died: 09-04-1902) 165

SECTION-J (167 to 168)
J-1 Dr. Jaisoorya, N.M. (Born: 26-09-1899 / Died: 1964) 168

SECTION-K (169 to 184)
K-1 Dr. Kent, Tyler (Born: 31-03-1849 / Died: 06-06-1916) 170

SECTION-L (185 to 188)
L-1 Dr. Lilienthal, Samuel (Born: 05-12-1815 / Died: 03-10-1891) 186

SECTION-M (189 to 206)
M-1 Dr. Majumdar, Jitendra Nath (Died: 30-11-1943) 190
M-2 Dr. Majumdar, Jnanendra Nath (Died: 15-09-1907 / Died: 29-11-1978) 191
M-3 Dr. Majumdar, Pratap Chandra (Died: 22-10-1922) 201
M-4 Dr. Mathur, K.N. (Born: 1906 / Died: 1977) 202
M-5 Dr. Mukherjee, A.N. (Died: 15-01-1954) 203
M-6 Dr. Mukherjee, Barid Baran (Born: 1873 / Died: 26-10-1940) 204
M-7 Dr. Muller, Father (Born: 13-03-1841 / Died: 01-11-1910) 205
M-8 Dr. Murty, V.R. (Born: 20-10-1904 / Died: 26-10-1940) 206

SECTION-N (207 to 209)
N-1 Dr. Nash, Eugene Beuharis (Born: 08-03-1838 / Died: 06-11-1917) 208
N-2 Dr. Nag, S.K. (Died: 22-03-1937) 209

SECTION-P (211 to 212)
P-1 Dr. Pillai, M.N. (Born: 04-04-1882 / Died: 1942) 212

SECTION-R (213 to 217)
R-1 Dr. Roberts, Herbert A. (Born: 07-05-1868 / Died: 13-10-1950) 214
R-2 Dr. Roy, V.M. Kulkarni (Born: 1908 / Died: 07-11-1965) 217

SECTION-S (219 to 256)
S-1 Dr. Sahni, B. (Born: 17-01-1925 / Died: 26-10-1997) 220
S-2 Dr. Sankaran, P. (Born: 15-11-1922 / Died: 20-01-1979) 225
S-3 Dr. Sarkar, B.K. (Born: 27-12-1901 / Died: 06-02-1981) 228
S-4 Dr. Schmidt, Pierre (Born: 22-07-1894 / Died: 15-10-1987) 235
S-5 Dr. Schuessler, Whilhelm Heinrich (Born: 21-08-1821 / Died: 30-03-1898) 237
S-6 Dr. Sen, Suresh Chandra (Born: 01-08-1880 / Died: 26-03-1968) 241
S-7 Dr. Sinha, G.N. (Died: 17-01-1959) 242
S-8 Dr. Sircar, Mahendra Lal (Born: 02-11-1883 / Died: 24-02-1904) 243

SECTION-T (257 to 264)
T-1 Dr. Trinks, Karl Friedrich (Born: 08-10-1800 / Died: 05-07-1868) 258
T-2 Dr. Tyler, Margaret Lucy (Born: 1857 / Died: 21-06-1943) 264

SECTION-Y (265 to 267)
Y-1 Dr. Yingling, William A. (Born: 12-01-1851 / Died: 03-04-1933) 266
Y-2 Dr. Younan, W. (Born: 1859 / Died: 23-10-1932) 267

A

SECTION-A .... Page 7 to 9

A-1 ***Dr. Allen, Henry C.***
(Born: 02-10-1830 / Died: 22-01-1909) 8

A-2 ***Dr. Allen, Timothy Field***
(Born: 24-04-1837 / Died: 05-12-1902) 9

Dr. Henry C. Allen

Born : 02-10-1830

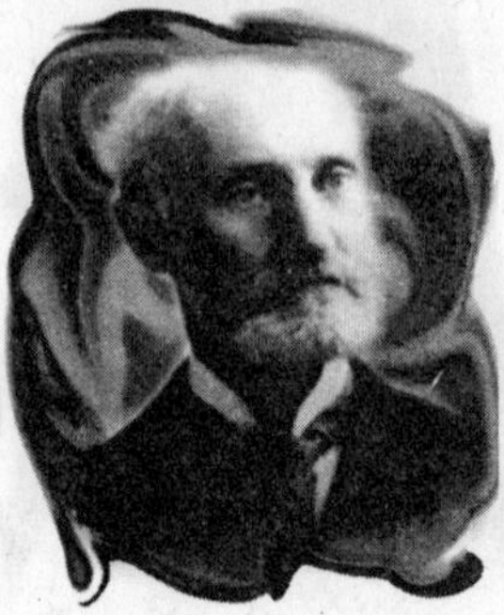

Died : 22-01-1909

Henry C. Allen, M.D., was born on the 2nd of October, 1830 in Brantford, Ontario, Canada. He studied medicine at the College of Physicians and Surgeons of Ontario, Completing his graduation in 1861. He studied homoeopathy at the Cleveland Homoeopathic College.

He served as a surgeon in the Civil War. After serving as a Civil War surgeon, he became professor of anatomy at the Cleveland Homoeopathic Medical College, and later at the Hahnemann College in Chicago. In the homoeopathic department of the university of Michigan at Ann Arbor, he was professor of materia medica and clinical medicine for five years, from 1880 to 1885.

He was the first dean and president of the governing board of the Hearing Medical College in Chicago. He was professor of materia media and teacher of the *organon* in the same college.

He was the editor and publisher of the *Medical Advance*. He also edited and partly rewrote the work of Dr. R.R. Lpregy on consumption. He added the section on the "Therapeutics of Consumption", and a repertory to Dr. Gregg's work, which was published under the title Gregy on Consumption, by Allen.

He authored many books: *Therapeutics of Intermittent Fever; Keynotes to the Leading Remedies of the Materia Medica; Materia Medica of the Nosodes* (issued after his death in 1910).

He was one of the founders of the IHA.

Section-A : Dr. Allen, Henry C.

Dr. Timothy Field Allen

Born : 24-04-1837

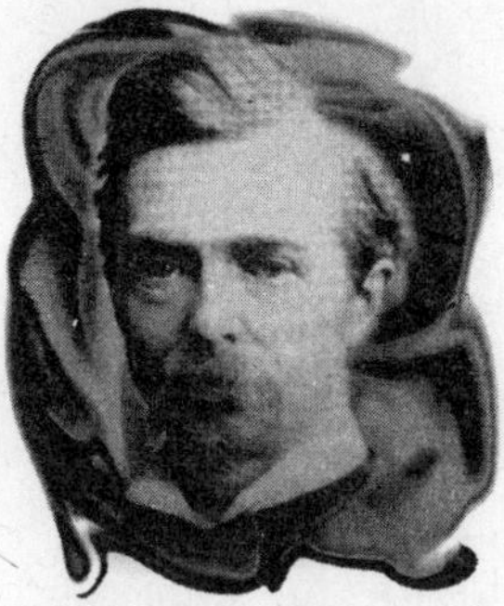

Died : 05-12-1902

Timothy Field Allen, M.D., was born on the 24th of April, 1837, in West Minster, Vermout. He received his early education at Amherst College and his medical degree from New York University.

He served as a surgeon in the civil war. He studied homoeopathy with Dr. P.P. Wells in Brooklyn, New York.

He was appointed as a professor of Materia Medica at the New York Homoeopathic Medical College. Later, he became president of the *same college. He was responsible for getting the half-million dollar grant from Rosewell P. Flower. This amount was used to build an addition to the college, which became the Flower Fifth Avenue Hospital.*

Allen worked as the Professor and Surgeon at New York Ophthalmic Hospital. He was responsible for converting it to a homoeopathic institution.

Music and botany were there two other areas of Allen's interest. He served as organist in several churches. He was on the Board of Directors of the New York Botanical Gardens.

He compiled the *Encyclopedia of Pure Materia Medica*. Its 10 volumes were published between 1874 and 1879. This Encylopedia was a complete record of all provings done with homoeopathic drugs.

Happiness is the innocent enjoyment of simple things.

SECTION-B .... Page 11 to 46

B-1 ***Dr. Banerjee, R.M.***
(Born: 28-11-1919 / Died: 09-04-1977) 12

B-2 ***Dr. Banerjee, Sripada*** (Died: 1966) 13

B-3 ***Dr. Bhatia, Anil***
(Born: 13-05-1942 / Died: 12-10-2002) 14

B-4 ***Dr. Boenninghausen, Clemens Maria Franz Von***
(Born: 12-03-1785 / Died: 26-01-1864) 17

B-5 ***Dr. Boericke, William***
(Born: 26-11-1849 / Died: 01-04-1929) 26

B-6 ***Dr. Boger, Cyrus Maxwell***
(Born: 13-05-1861 / Died: 02-09-1935) 28

B-7 ***Dr. Bose, B.K.***
(Born: 1879 / Died: 16-12-1977) 30

B-8 ***Dr. Burnett, James Compton***
(Born: 10-07-1840 / Died: 02-04-1901) 37

B-9 ***Dr. Byod, William Earnest***
(Born: 21-05-1891 / Died: 1955) 44

B-10 ***Dr. Bysack, Hem Chandra*** (Born: 1963) 46

Dr. R.M. Banerjee

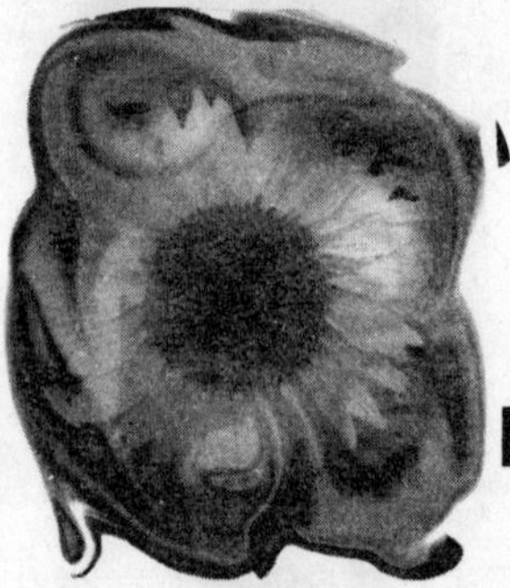

Born : 28-11-1919 **Died : 09-04-1977**

Dr. R. M. Banerjee was born on November 28, 1919 at Varanasi. He completed his school life in U.P., but at the sudden expiry of his father, had to start earning as a hawker.

After having attained some qualification in homoeopathic science he entered into practice in 1935 at Itawa in U.P.

In 1938 he joined the Second World War. During his army life, once he was court-martialled for protesting against British Government partially in privileges, which were withdrawn ultimately.

He also participated in anti-British Government activities and had been sent to jail.

He resigned from the army with six medals one 'Jangi Inam', as Viceroy's Commissioned officer in 1947.

He started homeopathic practice in Jabalpur in 1947-48. He was a strict and whole-hearted follower of Hahnemannin Homoeopathy. He, with his associates, formed a Homoeopathic Association at Jabalpur in 1962.

He was the founder father of Homoeopathic Medical College and Homoeopathic Medical Education in Jabalpur.

A man of strict discipline, punctuality, and hard workmanship departed from this world on April 9, 1977.

Section-B : Dr. Banerjee, R.M.

Dr. Sripada Banerjee

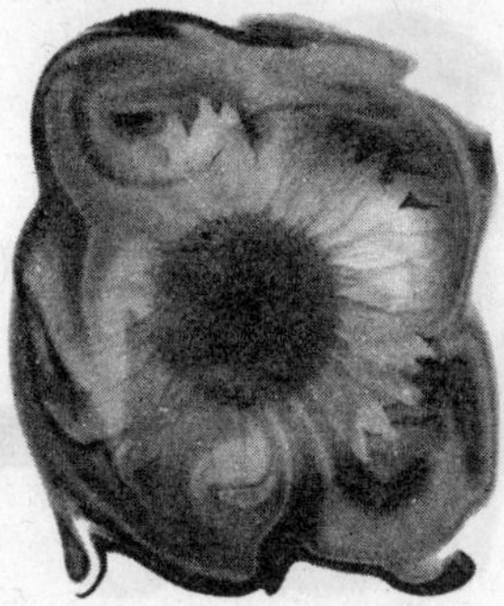

Died : 1966

Dr. Sripada Banerjee had his small homoeopathic dispensary in the Chandpole Bazar, Jaipur with a large clientele of patients and with a few disciples around him to assist. He was a liberal-minded person and, more or less, a routinist. He was responsible to a great extent in popularizing homoeopathy in Rajasthan and training up quite a good number of pupils. He practiced homoeopathy for a long period since 1930 till his death in October, 1966, at a ripe age.

Dr. Anil Bhatia

Born : 13-05-1942

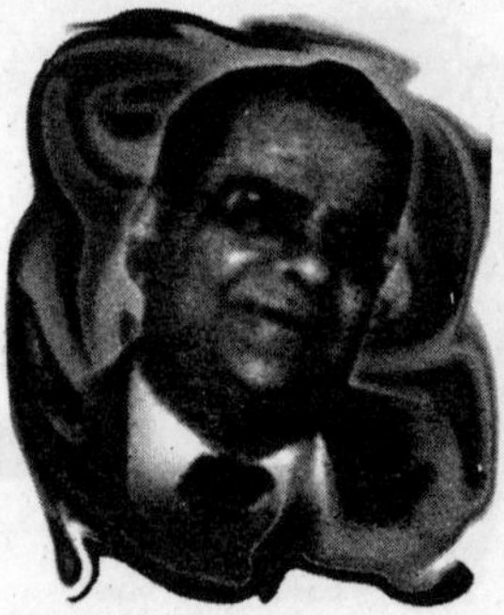

Died : 12-10-2002

Dr. Anil Bhatia expired on 12th Oct. 2002. The Homoeopathic fraternity has lost a very eminent homoeopath, well respected teacher, educator, leader, a dear friend and colleague to all.

Dr. Anil Bhatia had dedicated his entire lifetime for the upliftment of homoeopathy as a discipline.

Born on 13th May 1942, in Mandvi, Kutch, he completed his preliminary Homoeopathic education in 1962, Calcutta. The seeds of his belief in Homoeopathic system of medicine were sown then. Wanting to learn more about Homoeopathy as a science, not withstanding all financial and other difficulties he went to London's premier Homoeopathic Institute to obtain further qualifications - D.F. (Homoeopathic). In 1975 he completed M.B.S., Faculty of Homoeopathic Medicine, Calcutta.

After completing his education he started his private practice in Calcutta. But his vision at that young age was to create a uniform educational regulation for homoeopathic education.

His dedication for Homoeopathy was seen early on when he left a flourishing private practice, and even as a young doctor who had returned after obtaining a coveted degree from London, he still decided to move to Savli, a small village near Baroda. He was offered the post of "Principal" at the Homoeopathic College in Savli (1971-1975). This event can be considered as a turning point in his life when he found the path to achieve his goals for educational reforms in Homoeopathy.

From 1975-1986 he was the Principal of Chandaben Mohanbhai Patel Homoeopathic Medical College, Mumbai. Under his leadership and interaction with the University of Mumbai, Central Council of

Homoeopathy and other such organizations, he was able to introduce the first B.H.M.S. course in India, a recognized degree course from University of Mumbai.

Dr. Bhatia made a lot of contributions towards the fields of Education and Research in Homoeopathy. As a Chairman of Eduction Committee of Central Council of Homoeopathy. During his tenure uniform educational regulations for homoeopathic education were formulated and implemented in universities and boards of homoeopathy all over the country. Also with his guidance, Post Graduate Course in homoeopathic medicine (M.D. Hom.) were introduced for the first time in the country, in 1989-1990. Over the years, he developed various homoeopathic colleges and hospitals in accordance to norms laid down by the Central Council of Homoeopathy.

Dr. Bhatia held various positions of leadership through which he was able to bring very significant reforms in Homoeopathic education and research at the national level. He was appointed Honorary Advisor, Homoeopathy, Ministry of Health and Family Welfare; Member, Governing Body & Scientific Advisory Committee - Central Council for Research in Homoeopathy; Chairman, Academic Committee, National Institute of Homoeopathy.

As the Chairman of Homoeopathic Committee for Drugs and Technical Advisory Board, Ministry of Health, Govt. of India and Chairman, Homoeopathic Pharmacopeia Committee, Govt. of India, he strived to bring quality control and standardization in Homoeopathic Therapeutics.

A part of Dr. Bhatia's vision was to bring recognition and acclaim to the discipline of Homoeopathy around the world. He was selected as the official delegated by the Govt. of India for the International Homoeopathic Congress at Washington D.C., U.S.A. He attended the conference of Organization of Homoeopathic Medical International in Mexico where he received International Award of Merit - for his contributions to Homoeopathy. He was a speaker at the conference of "Liga International Homoeopathic League" at Seattle. He was also invited as a Guest Lecturer at George Vithoulkas International School of Homoeopathy, Athens, Greece in 1998 and to School of Homoeopathy, Krakow, Poland in 1999.

Dr. Anil Bhatia had a very successful private practice, and his clinical experience stretched over 40 yrs. His ability of listen and understand his patients, his razor sharp clinical acumen, his knowledge of Homoeopathic Philosophy and Therapeutics, and his transparent honesty in his limitations won him the trust of hundreds of patients and doctors (both homoeopathic and allopathic) alike. Inspite of busy practice, he opted to serve as Honorary Homoeopathic Physician at B.N. Nanavati Hospital, Mumbai where he would see patients from all strata of society.

As a token of all his achievement, he received the Homoeo Dynasty Great Masters Award in 1995, and was the recipient of Dr. Hahnemann Memorial National Award in 1999.

The complete list of his awards and achievements are very exhaustive to list here, but for Dr. Anil Bhatia – the most satisfying and rewarding thing in life was to have been able to give a large part of himself to others – to Homoeopathic education, research, and to most of all, his patients.

Dr. Clemens Maria Franz Von Boenninghausen

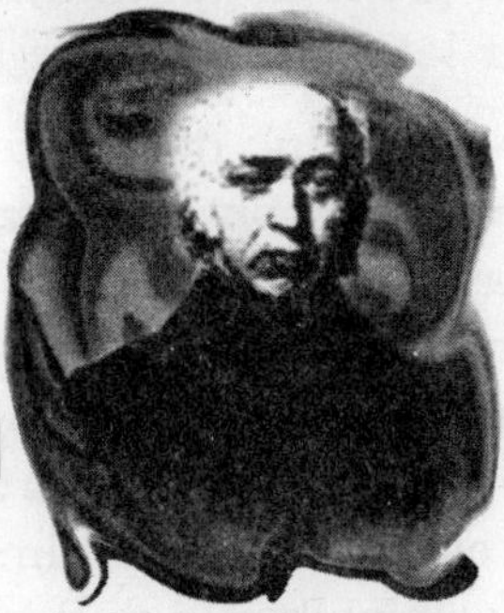

Born : 12-03-1785 **Died : 26-01-1864**

There must be something in it — This is often the first germ which breaks through the smooth surface of traditional conviction. The doctor, we are taught, takes illness away, subconsciously we know, of course, he might take our appendix away, but the illness he suppresses. However, that is quite correct, 'everybody' says so, and 'everybody' is invariably right. Until one day the doctor fails to suppress whatever is ailing us, and we accept, smiling with incredulity but desperately anxious to be rid of our complaint, the advice of 'Like Cures Like'. Success begets doubt — is there something in it, after all? We study the principle, become convinced, converted and enthusiastic". The history of Homoeopathy is abound with such instances.

The narrative on this leaf from our past history glitters with the glory of the life, dedication and contributions to Homoeopathy of Dr. Clemens Maria Franz Von Boenninghausen whom the ordains of destiny had imparted all virtues to be exceptional, excellent and high in whatever field of activities he decided to take interest. Exactly a hundred and sixty two years ago, Clemens Maria Franz Von Boenninghausen, the late 'Officer of Justice' to his Royal Highness, Louis Napoleon of Holland, lay on his sick-bed and the attending physicians did not know what to do with him. The disease they declared to be suppurative phthisis, Von Boenninghausen, hardly more than 40 years old, suffered exceedingly and believed his death to be near. The doctors concurred. It may well to that the patient listened to the suggestion of his friend, the botanist and homoeopathic physician, Dr. Weihe, of Hervorden (Westphalia), because he was apathetically convinced that he could not get worse any way and might as well give those funny little pills a trial. The selection of the remedy was made on the basis of a report on his illness which Von Boenninghausen himself had complied in great detail and, apparently, with great accuracy and half a year later he was hale and hearty once more.

The attitude of his allopathic doctors seems to have puzzled Von Boenninghausen considerably. Naturally he had told them how his life had been saved, he had generously offered the secret which would lead to similar successes in their own practice - but was refused, politely and otherwise. Westphalian people are said to be strong-headed. The refusal, but, strengthened Von Boenninghausen's interest and made him determined to learn more about this therapy which could pull him back into life when others had given him up as lost. His intensive studies resulted, apart from many books and treatises, in the final decision to become a homoeopathic physician himself and to bring to others the services of this revolutionary therapy from which he had so greatly benefitted.

THE ANCESTORS & THE FAMILY

His father, Ludwing Ernst Von Boenninghausen, a Lieutenant Colonel and Chamberlain of the Prince of Munster and a Knight of the Dutch order, died on May 5th, 1812. His mother, Theresia, who was the Baroness of Weichs on Wenne, died on April 7th, 1828. He had five brothers and sisters, only one of whom was elder to him, and one was a half-brother. The name and coat of arms of his ancestors can be traced upto the 13th Century, and one of whom an Austrian General Field Marshal was made a Baron of Westphalia and Rhineland on the 26th of May, 1632. Nearly all of the Boenninghausens devoted themselves to the military career.

BIRTH & CHILDHOOD

He was born on the 12th of March, 1785 at Heringhaven, an estate in overyssel, a province of the Netherlands. This estate belonged to his father.

EDUCATION

In his early life Boenninghausen lived in countryside and his body was well-developed due to riding, swimming, hunting and other physical exercises but his education could not develop in the same proportion. At the age of 12 years he came to the gymnasium (High School) in Munster. He was found to be amongst the most uninformed students and was allotted a seat on last benches but he worked his way up even in the first term and continued to hold it.

After attending the school for six years at Munster, Boenninghausen, at the age of 18 yrs. entered the Dutch University of Groningen where he studied law as well as natural history and medicine. On 30th of August, 1806, he received the degree of *Doctor Utrinsque Juris* and on the 1st of October; the same year he was appointed lawyer at the Supreme Court at Deventer. Louis Bonaparte, the king of Holland, appointed him as an Auditor to the Privy Council. Within a year he was promoted to the post of Auditor to the King and within fourteen days of this appointment he was made the General Secretary des requettes. He was given responsibilities of the Royal Librarian and Chief of the Topographical Bureau. He remained in Holland and worked on these burdensome posts until the resignation of the King of Holland on the 1st of July, 1810. Boenninghausen was severally grieved by this resignation and refused all employment in the Dutch Civil Service. In September, 1810, he returned to his paternal estate and devoted time to his favourite subject.

He was married in the autumn of 1812 and went to his ancestral estate of Darup in Westphalia. There he started to develop the resources of the estate and started correspondence with the important agriculturists of Germany like Thaer and Schwers. He wrote many articles for the famous journal of agriculture and botany, 'MAEGLINSCHE ANNALEN'. His article 'THE CULTURE OF RYE ACCORDING TO TWENT' received wide acclaim. A separate issue of the journal was issued for this article. He was the founder of the Agricultural Society for the District of Munster. In 1816 he was appointed as the President of the Provincial Court of Justice for the Westphalia district in Oesfield and worked until 1822. He was also made the Joint Commissar for the registration of surveyed lands. He published his famous book 'Statistics of Westphalia Agriculture', in 242 pages. His position called for many conferences. Thus he got ample opportunities to travel and to compile his 'PRODOMUS FLORAE MONASTERIENSIS', published in 1824, dealing with the floral riches of the provinces. He was made Director and given charge of the Botanical Gardens of Munster and came in contact with the great botanists of Europe.

He was honoured by the botanists C. Sprengel and Reichenbach, Sprengel in his book SYSTEMA VEGETABILIS (Volume III, P. 245) and Reichanback in his UEBERS' DES GEMWAECHSTEICHS, (P. 197) named a genus of plants after him. He was honoured by the Honorary Degrees of many respected societies.

CONVERSION TO HOMOEOPATHY

In the fall of 1827 he became seriously ill and was diagnosed to be suffering from purulent tuberculosis, which took a serious turn by the spring of 1828 and all hopes of recovery were given up. Boenninghausen wrote a farewell letter to his friend of botany, Dr. A. Weihe, M.D., of Hervorden. Weihe was the first homoeopathic physician in the whole of the provinces of Rhineland and Westphalia although Boenninghausen was ignorant of it. Dr. Weihe requested an exact and detailed description of the disease and its concomitants and expressed the hope that he may get well. Boenninghausen complied the symptoms in great detail and with great accuracy. Weihe prescribed *Pulsatilla* for Boenninghausen who gradually recovered and by the summer he was cured of his ailment. This was a turning point in the life of Boenninghausen and in the course of homoeopathy in Germany and that part of Europe. Boenninghausen became a firm believer and ardent promoter of homoeopathy. He was able to convert, to homoeopathy, Dr. Lutterback and Dr. Tuisting. His influence, help and teaching brought many new adherents to homoeopathy in the countries like France, Holland, America, etc. By a Royal order dated July 11th, 1843 of King Friedrich Wilhelm IV, he was empowered to practice medicine. He completed his job of land registry and resigned from Dutch Civil Service to devote whole-heartedly to the practice of homoeopathy.

Boenninghausen was in regular correspondence with Hahnemann and his disciples like Stapf, Gross, Muehlenbein, Weihe and other 'Veterana of the old Guard'.

In 1848 he founded the SOCIETY OF THE HOMOEOPATHIC PHYSICIANS of Westphalia and the Rhineland and started yearly assembly of the homoeopathic physicians of the region. He was honoured with the membership of most of the existing homoeopathic societies. The Cleveland Homoeopathic Medical College (North America) made him MEDICINAE DOCTORIS by a diploma on the 1st of March, 1854. The Emperor of France appointed him as "Knight of the Legion of Honour" on April 20, 1861.

DEMISE

Boenniaghausen remained physically sound and mentally active till his very old age. In the winter of 1863 he suffered from bronchial catarrh but he continued to attend to his afternoon calls. On January 22nd, he completed his written work after a walk. On 24th of January, 1864 he suffered from a stroke of apoplexy and paralysis of left side and died on 26th January, 1864 at 3.45 A.M. at the age of seventy-eight years 10 months and 14 days. On his death the obituary in ALLGEMEINE HOMOEO-PATHISCHE ZEITUNG wrote:

"Our science has lost in him one of its first leaders, our journal one of its best co-laborers, the society of the Physicians of the Rhineland and Westphalia its head and its pillar, or Central Society a much honoured member, and we, personally - a faithful friend and loving teacher."

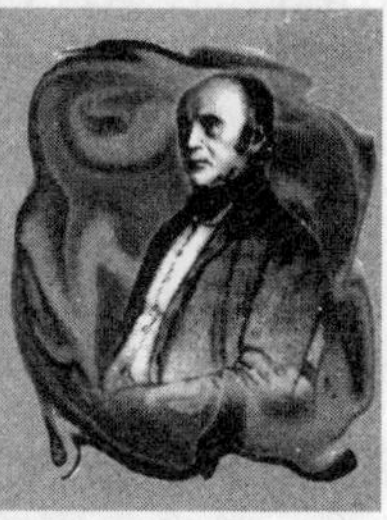

HOMOEOPATHY IN THE FAMILY

Out of his seven sons two followed his example. His first Son, Karl (Born on 5th of November, 1826), started living at Paris and was married to the adopted daughter of Hahnemann's second wife Madame Melanie. He settled down in Paris and practiced homoeopathy in conjunction with madame Hahnemann. He died on the 13th July, 1902 while his wife (Hahnemann's adopted daughter) had died 3 years earlier, i.e. on the 7th of February, 1899. Boenninghausen's second son, Friedrich (Born on April 14, 1828) adopted a legal career but after passing the first two state examinations he began to study medicine, at the age of 27 years. He was very delicate in childhood and suffered from blindness for two years. He was cured by his father and he did not use glasses even in his old age. After studying medicine for 4 years in Bonn and Berlin and passing medical examination he settled in 1859 as an assistant to his father.

He remained in his paternal home for more than fifty years and was quite famous as a homoeopathic physician. After a short illness, he died on the 6th of August, 1910 at the age of 83 years.

HIS CONTRIBUTIONS

About him it was written:

"...........and if we view his life and consider with what excellent qualities and virtues it was equipped, the constant activity in the endeavour to benefit his fellow man and posterity, surely, the all-consuming death cannot wipe out his life, for it will live in the history of our science, it will continue to be a glorious example for our young men ...."

H.A. Roberts wrote: "The works of Boeninghausen are among the most comprehensive in logic, philosophy and applicability of the early writers — perhaps with the single exception of the works of Hahnemann. The most comprehensive and far reaching in influence."

He says further: "It was Boenninghausen who first evaluated remedies in relation to the individual symptoms, and it was he who first introduced various other methods of relationship of any given remedy to the individual case."

About his another contribution of much greater value, Boger says, "Boenninghausen's analytical mind evolved the doctrine of concomitants, which has been all too often overlooked."

Boenninghausen's contribution in the field of Repertory has been acclaimed by all. Boger writes:

"With the possible exception of Jahr, Boenninghausen was the first to recognise the value and necessity of some form of index to the rapidly growing list of remedies being developed and proven by Hahnemann and his disciples. There is same question whether or not Boenninghausen was actually the first to produce such an index or repertory, it has been substantiated, however, that in the early 1830's Boenninghausen produced such a volume in printed form, and that Boenninghausen's first volume of repertory index was evaluated by means of different styles or type while Jahr's first index was not. Hahnemann at first used Jahr's compilation, but shortly gave it up in favour of Boenninghausen's repertory. Boenninghausen's REPERTORY OF THE ANTIPSORICS is the great progenitor of the repertories we have today."

His THERAPEUTIC POCKET BOOK was the result of the attempt to produce concise and comprehensive index.

T.L. Bradford wrote:

"No oneman, except Hahnemann left so deep an impression

upon the literature of homoeopathy, or has exerted so great an influence in favour of the homoeopathy taught by Hahnemann, as Boenninghausen."

He devoted himself especially to presenting the materia medica so that the chief characteristics of each remedy might be thoroughly understood by the practitioners and his writings are mostly devoted to that object.

Most of the systematic works written by Boenninghausen concerning homoeopathy were published between 1928 and 1846.

He was a constant contributor between 1828 to 1846, to homoeopathic journals like ARCHIV FUER HOMOEOPATHISCHE HEILKUNST, ALLGEMEINE HOMOEOPATHISCHE ZEITUNG, etc.

H.A. Roberts explains Boenninghausen's contribution regarding his system of analogy in these words:

"Boenninghausen comprehended the difficulties encountered by the physician in securing a complete picture of the case, and his comparisons of his case records and the records of provers convinced him that the same lack of observation existed in the provers as existed in patients.

Noting these deficiencies in the materia medica, therefore, and realizing the importance of these auxiliary, modifying and concomitant symptoms of disease, Boenninghausen for many years diligently observed and collected all such symptoms as they appeared in the cases which came to him for treatment. Every case was examined symptomatically with this purpose always in view, viz., to make every symptom as complete in itself as possible, covering the specific points of locality, sensation, conditions of aggravation and amelioration, and the concomitance of co-existence of other symptoms under the same circumstances.

He soon learned that symptoms which existed in an incomplete state in some part of a given case could be reliably completed by analogy, by observing the conditions of other parts of the case. If, for instance, it was not possible by questioning a patient to decide what aggravated or ameliorated a particular symptom of the case, the patient would readily express a condition of amelioration of some other symptoms. It did not take long to discover that conditions of aggravation or amelioration are not confined to this or that particular symptom, but that, like the red thread in the cordage of the British Navy, they apply to all the symptoms of the case.

Boenninghausen tells in his preface: "From one point of view the indicated conditions of aggravation or amelioration have a far more significant relation to the totality of the case and to its single symptoms than is usually supposed, they are never confined exclusively to one or another symptom, but, on the contrary, a correct choice of the suitable remedy depends very often chiefly upon them."

HOMOEOPATHIC WRITINGS

1831 : The Cure of Cholera and its Preventives.

1832 : Repertory of the Antipsoric Medicines.

1833 : Summary View of the Chief Sphere of Operation of the Antipsoric Remedies and their Characteristic Peculiarities, as an appendix to their repertory.

An attempt at a Homoeopathic Therapy of Intermittent Fever. Contributions to a knowledge of the Peculiarities of Homoeopathic Remedies.

1834 : Homoeopathy, a Manual for the Non-medical Public.

1835 : Repertory of Non-Antipsoric remedies.

1836 : Attempt at Showing the Relative Kinship of Homoeopathic Medicines.

1845 : Essay on the Homoeopathic Treatment of Intermittent Fevers. (Translated and edited by Charles Julius Hempel) P. 56.

1846 : Therapeutic Manual for Homoeopathic Physicians.

1847 : Therapeutic Pocket Book for Homoeopathists, to be used at the bedside of the patient, and in the study of the Materia Medica, P. 483 (This book contains concordance of homoeopathic remedies).

1849 : Brief instruction for Non-physicians as to the Prevention and Cure of Cholera.

1853 : The Two Sides of the Human Body and their Relationships.

1854 : The Sides of the Body and Drug Affinities, Homoeopathic Exercises. pp. 28.

1860 : The Homoeopathic Treatment of Whooping Cough in its Various Forms.

1863 : The Aphorisms of Hippocrates, with notes by a Homoeopathic Pocket Book for Homoeopathic Physicians.

1870 : The Homoeopathic Treatment of Wooping Cough, pp. 199.

1873 : Homoeopathic Therapia of Intermittent and other Fevers, p. 243.

1891 : Therapeutic Pocketbook for Homoeopathic Physicians, to be used at the Bedside, and in the study of the Materia Medica. A new American Edition, by Timothy Field Allen. pp. 484. (In this edition the new American Remedies were included. The index to this book was printed after the book was issued, and placed in the copies as they were sold.)

1908 : Lesser Writings, p. 358, B. & T. Indian prints of this book is available. It contains articles written by Boenninghausen and published in contemporary journals.

SOURCE MATERIALS ON BOENNINGHAUSEN

1. Kleinert : Geshichte der Homoeopathic, p-130-134.
2. Lute's Fl. Blatter, February, 24, 1864.
3. Medical counsellor, Vol. 11, P. 492.
4. Allgemeine Homoeopathis she Zeitung, Volume 68, P. 16.
5. American Homoeopathic Review, Volume 4, P. 433.
6. World's Congress, Volume 2, P. 36.
7. British Homoeopathic Journal, Volume 22, P. 351
8. Repou : Histoire de la Medicale Homoeopathique, Volume 2.
9. Indo-German Homoeopathic Review , Volume III, No. 3. 91, 348/91.
10. Kanjilal, Dr. J.N. : Clemens Maria Franz Von Boenninghausen: Homoeo Jyoti, 1965-66.

Dr. William Boericke

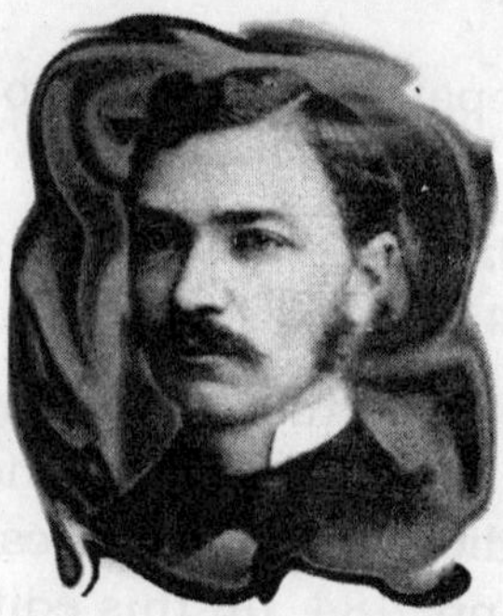

Born : 26-11-1849 **Died : 01-04-1929**

William Boericke, M.D., was born in Austria on 26th of the November, 1849. When he was a child he went to the United States and settled in Ohio. In 1880, he attended (entered) the medical school and graduated from Hahnemann Medical College in Philadelphia.

In 1870 he went to California to manage the Boericke and Tafel Pharmacy in San Francisco. He set up a successful practice in San Francisco.

He was one of the founders of the Homoeopathic Medical College of San Francisco. He wrote "Boericke's Materia Medica" in 1901. The book went through nine editions in his lifetime. Oscar, Boerick's brother and a graduate of Hahnemann Medical College, added a repertory to the book in 1906.

Boericke served in the faculty of Hahnemann Medical College in San Francisco and worked as an editor for *The California Homoeopath*. His son, Garth Wilkinson Boericke, followed his footsteps and became a homoeopath. He introduced *Hecla Lava* into the Boerick's Materia Medica. Jean Barnard, his grand-daughter, recalls: "He used to call all us kids *'Done'* and he would always kiss and hug us, he was a very loving man."

"Our family belonged to the high society in San Francisco at that time because Grand dad was the physician of choice in the area between 1880 and 1920. People came from all over the world to be treated homoeopathically by him. My parents used to say 'Poor Papa' because he worked so hard, and the thing I remember the most is them saying 'don't bother Papa'. My family was very devoted to him, whatever he said was the law. Although he emigrated from Austria, he had no accent and there was no German spoken in our house. He and I used to go on walks together down Tamalpais Avenue. I remember he took such long steps, I would scurry along next to him as he engaged me in conversation."

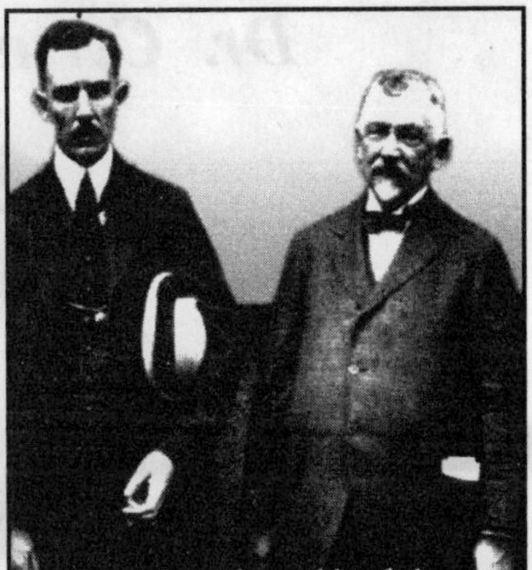
Garth Boericke and his father, William Boericke, 1927

Boericke died on April 1, 1929 due to a heart attack.

His granddaughter recalls, "Many months before, he had developed angina symptoms after racing my father down Tamalpais Avenue. He was about 5'9" and fairly fast on his feet for a man in his late 70s."

Boericke's house caught fire two months after his death and everything was turned to ash except all of his homoeopathic books and the stone fire place.

Dr. Cyrus Maxwell Boger

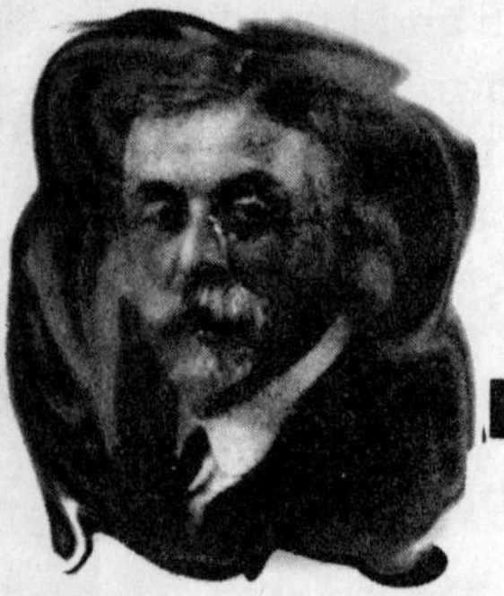

Born : 13-05-1861 **Died : 02-09-1935**

Cyrus Maxwell Boger M.D., was born on the 13th of May, 1861, in Western Pennsylvania.

Boger was a German Scholar. He graduated from the Philadelphia College of Pharmacy. In 1888, he received his medical degree from Hahnemann College, in Philadelphia.

He worked as the president of IHA in 1904. He translated "Boenninghausen's Characteristics and Repertory" into the English language in 1905. He made additions to the Kent's repertory and published them along with a table of times of amelioration and aggravation, and a proving of Samarskite.

In 1915, he wrote a book, named "Synoptic Key and Repertory". In 1931 *he developed the Boger General Analysis and Card Repertory,* which went through several editions. This repertory consists of about 360 cards and each card represents a rubric. If a remedy is indicated for the rubric, a hole is punched in the card in the appropriate place. Simply pull the cards, *arrange them in a pile, and then look for the holes that go all the way through.*

Boger's repertory is an eliminative repertory therefore the first card must be an accurate symptom of the case. He suggests to use the Card Repertory to find the general symptoms of the case, while the Kent Repertory should be used for the specific symptoms of the case.

From 1924 until his death he was in the faculty of the AFH postgraduate course.

"Boger uses Electrical Potentizer to make higher potency of a

---

Section-B : Dr. Boger, Cyrus Maxwell

remedy. Electrical potencies were made on a machine, constructed by Dr. Skcle's son, of Chicago. Boger has this machine in his office and he personally operates it." Now, the whereabouts of this machine are unknown.

Boger died at the age of 74 on the 2nd of September, 1935. He died from food poisoning after eating a tin of home-pressured tomatoes. He was always fond of home-canned foods.

Dr. B.K. Bose

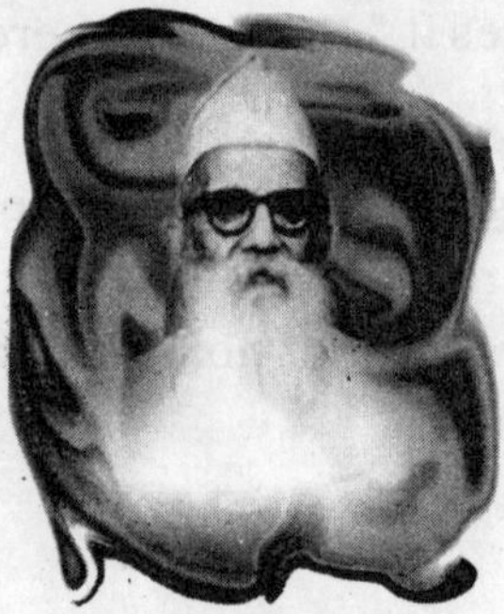

Born : 1879 **Died : 16-12-1977**

The bearded saint-looking gentleman who walks erect, travels everyday in trams and buses at peak office hours rush, has a voice which usually needs no mike in any meeting or gathering, is above eighty years in age and he is Dr. B.K. Bose, the only living student of immortal Kent in this part of globe.

He was born in 1879. His father was an Additional Judge and so he had all that is known as respectable family, luxurious life and elated environment. But it was a period when Indian nationalism was awakening itself from a slumberous sleep of foreign domination and a bright hope of independent India was dawning on this vast continent. Bengal, the undivided Bengal, was the seat of greatest turbulence and political unrest.

British Government wanted to cow down the independent spirit of Bengal and so the conspiracy of 'partition of Bengal' was hatched. Bengal fought to its fame and Bijoy Kumar Bose joined the movement whole heartedly. He considered it to be his personal war.

The boy whom the family and the parents wanted to be an I.C.S. became a rebel, and under-ground terrorist, an absconder. He wanted to over-throw the empire whom his family wanted him to serve.

To avoid arrest, to learn the advanced techniques of manufacturing hand-grenades and to acquire arms for struggle, he fled to France with great difficulties, with no money.

The British Govt. pressed the French Govt. for his arrest and extradition and the same story of 'hunt and run' started in France. He had to leave France with the help of some local Indians and

---

Section-B : Dr. Bose, B.K.

French sympathisers of Indian freedom movement. U.S.A. was his next destination.

Local authorities in U.S.A. wanted to know the object of his sojourn. Explanations were unsatisfactory. Pressure started mounting. He took admission into New York Homoeopathic Medical College and Flower Hospital as a cover. But the place had no utility for his main objective. He shifted to Ann Arbor, and entered the University of Michigan. Two years he was there studying 'non violence' in a recognised university and 'violence' in the shadowy underworld. He came in contact with Dr. Dewey, Smith, etc. Dewey directed him to J.T. Kent in Hering Medical College.

He was granted an interview with the Dean.

The Dean was an interesting gentleman. He asked "Well, Bose, you want to take admission in Homoeopathic Department?" "Yes Sir!" was the prompt but humble reply. "Is Homoeopathy recognised in your country?" "No, Sir!" calm admission of a fact. "Will you get any service when you go there after obtaining homoeopathic degree?"

"No Sir," the same obedient humble voice.

"Then you must be a damn fool to study this Science which has no service, no recognition, no future for you."

The inside rebel took charge. No more calm voice, no more obedient humbleness. The sharp voice came like the crash of a whip. "And Sir! you must be a greater fool teaching students who have no scope or future in their countries and your Govt. must be the greatest of all foolish Governments granting passports and visas to such students. You were slaves, we are slaves, you are independent and we will be independent. The students of independent India will not come to study Homoeopathy here, they shall have their own college." This story was narrated by the Dean in the farewell speech to graduating students in which there were two more Indian students. Kent heard his story, gave a friendly smile and a fatherly pat and took him into Hering Homoeopathic Medical College.

It was Kent who transformed this rebel into a Homoeopath, this anarchist into a healer of human sufferings. The non-violence of reasoning and understanding won over the violence of youth and immaturity. The desire to change by force surrendered before the will to serve; the political agitator and worker became a humanist, a physician. Bijoy Kumar Bose became a medical graduate.

The environment there was genuine, homoeopathic and scholarly. He came in contact with Dr. William Tod Helmuth, J.H. Allen, H.C. Allen and a host of others. Sir John Weir of Royal Homoeopathic Hospital, London, was an outgoing student then.

Finally, he took admission into Kansas City University and received his Master's degree. There he studied Osteopathy too and obtained D.O. (i.e. Diploma in Osteopathy).

His return to India was possible only due to personal connections and influence of Dr. Kent.

Dr. B.K. Bose, M.D., D.O., started his practice in Calcutta with Dr. D.N. Ray and Younan. The soft-spoken, shy, introvert, handsome convinced Kentian young homoeopath with elite habits and aristocratic choice for things was invited to Banaras by some eminent political leaders. He started his practice there and became family physician of Shri Moti Lal Nehru. It was there that he established a lucrative practice and visited the Maharajas of India and its neighbouring countries on professional calls. It was a life of service, fame and luxury.

Dr. D.N. Ray, the Founder and Principal of Calcutta Homoeopathic Medical College was growing old and he was anxious about the future of the institution. He knew B.K. Bose and remembered him.

Those old observing and experienced, eyes of Dr. Ray could see the selfless and non-attached worker behind that fashionable and aristocratic exterior of Bose. He was right. Dr. Bose served the institution for forty years without any big post though he was the senior most member of the staff.

In that luxury-seeking exterior Dr. Ray could see the soul of duty and service who can go to the extreme limit of personal sacrifice. Dr. Bose was giving usual lectures in the classes and rounds in the wards only 3 hours after the death of his only son.

And in that calm and serene, soft and shy exterior, Dr. Ray could see a fighter with a strong vertebral column who can stand firm while opposing the wrong or while being opposed on a right cause. He was right again. Dr. Bose has always stood against what he has considered to be wrong whether in State Homoeopathic

Faculty or in Association meeting or in the College or Government attitudes. He opposed his own friends whom he brought, converted to homoeopathy, gave post and power and whom he obeyed for long forty years. His own intimate friend he opposed with thunderous voice and with tearful eyes, when the welfare of the institution demanded it. He remained firm when all the students of the college took mass transfer certificate and joined another college started by some of the members of the staff.

Dr. Ray wrote a personal letter to Dr. Bose insisting his return to Calcutta and begging this personal sacrifice of him. To Dr. Ray it was a choice which was to prove its justification in future but to Dr. Bose it was an immediate call of obligation to the science, the profession and the teachers, a call of duty to the science of whose efficacy and truth he was convinced.

Who knows the torrents of thoughts which might have overflooded him? All that he had earned, the money, the fame, the reputation was to remain and he was to start again his practice, his life, his circle. He was to leave behind everything which a man craves for. He made a decision and he has never regretted it. He came to Calcutta and joined Calcutta Homoeopathic Medical College.

Nearly half of a century has passed. The handsome youth with aristocratic habits has changed into a saintly old savant. The rebellious heart has given place to a sentimental Godly-heart who thinks for masses, feels for sick and cries for poor.

The Calcutta Homoeopathic Medical College has grown up. The hut is replaced by a palacial building of 3 blocks. The five-bedded hospital is now a 200 bedded hospital with 10 wards. The old pals and colleagues have retired, have departed one by one. The new blood, the new appointments, the new staff is filling the vacant chairs. His routine is same, the routine which has been followed with clock like regularity of coming every day at 9.30 a.m., attending to out-door patients, indoor patients, giving lectures in the classes, etc.

The history of Indian homoeopathy will be incomplete without Calcutta Homoeopathic Medical College and on the chapter on Calcutta Homoeopathic Medical College some name shall shine prominently, the most prominent and bold of which shall be that of Dr. Bose, Dr. B.K. Bose. Every brick and stone shall testify to his endowments, his services and his individual role in the step by step, stage by stage, extension, progress and development of this institution, the oldest in India, the biggest in Asia, the only in world today. When he joined it was weak, indistinct and gasping, when he retires he shall leave behind the greatest institution in regard to building, staff, teaching and record of purity of purpose.

To the world of homoeopathy, he and Sir John Weir are the last two living students of Kent, Allen and Helmuth.

To the Indian homoeopathy, he is the symbol of pure Hahnemanian and Kentian Homoeopathy and the last pillar of that generation of giant homoeopaths, whom India particularly Bengal had the unique fortune of witnessing.

To the West Bengal homoeopathy, he is a temple where homoeopathic practitioners and students of world have poured in to learn, to express faith and devotion, to show reverence and to bow head.

To the Calcutta Homoeopathic Medical College, he is the source of nutrition and energy. He is a good teacher, a considerate boss, and a complaint register of everyone, for everything, everyday.

To his past students, he is the light, the guide, the spirit and the evergreen memory of a whip which will not let them falter, will not let them deviate and will not let them submit or surrender.

To his present students he is a good-hearted tyrant, a loving father who has well disciplined mind but rough tongue, a person who remembers their family matters and conditions but pretends extreme forgetfulness and carelessness.

Out of nearly 643 teachers employed in recognised and non-recognised homoeopathic institutions of India, 481 are his students who write to him regularly and this is his achievement.

He has proved that a Homoeopathic Hospital of this magnitude can exist at a nominal or at times without any monetary help from Governments, and this is his achievement.

All his life he has fought, as an underground terrorist against mighty British empire, as a practitioner of a non-recognised system against the State and the Central Governments, as puritan and Hahnemanian homoeopath against the neo-homoeopaths and so called modernists, as a protestor of his institution against the power corrupt post mongers and as a saviour of the *under-dogs* against the wrath of vindictive and revengeful OVER-LORDS of this science.

Section-B : Dr. Bose, B.K.

And his achievement is that he has remained alone and alone, and alone. He belongs to no party, no association, and to no group.

His only fault is that he fears none, conspires against no body, wants no publicity, talks no pleasing language. And that is why he is misunderstood, and he is deserted and alone. Probably he prefers it the way it is.

His only fault is that he attends no conference, sings no songs of self – praise, boasts of no cures, writes no book by copying *head of one* and *tail of another* of old classics, narrates no painted stories of his services and sacrifices and that is why his name is not printed and that is why he is not publicised and that is why he is not the Chairman of any Government appointed committee. Probably he prefers it the way it is.

His greatest fault is that he has secluded himself in the thought and works of the development of Calcutta Homeopathic Medical College, in serving the suffering masses who throng him in hundreds every day. He is the straight forward person of principle who believes more in practice than preaching and that is why he is misunderstood as arrogant, obstinate, orthodox and unpredictable and probably he prefers it too that way.

THE SICKNESS

The news of the sickness of Dr. B.K. Bose, the homoeopath, the teacher, the guide and the light of thousands of young men and women reached everywhere and his devotees and students came to see their master. On 28-11-77, in the evening, I asked "why don't you get well?" His answer was, "I will not". I was equally blunt, "why don't you die than?" "I will die, but not now". "Then what are you doing? Suffering and making others suffer?" "No, No, it is not suffering. I am tasting death. I am watching how slowly death comes and life departs. I see that death is gradually occupying the areas of my life vacated by the life in me. There is total disobedience, organs are not obeying me, mind is only obeying in part. Accidental death are sudden. Gradual death is by increasing disobedience of organs and body." Then I remembered that he had wanted to taste death before dying. In one of the condolence meeting this was the type of death he preferred.

THE DEPARTURE

Somewhere in a very rhythmical and well-modulated voice

was heard AZAN for the Namaz of Asar. The winter sun was setting early and the evening was hurrying to meet the day. The Azan was a call to prayer and to bandagi to God.

The life was leaving the body of this material world for an unknown world. The activities of the whole days were coming to a final close. Dr. B.K. Bose was leaving us and at 4.22 p.m. surrounded by his students, his relatives, neighbours, some of his patients he departed. He left his deeds to be remembered, his example to be emulated, his activities to be worshipped and his footsteps to be followed. Some one said,

The Nature shall rise and say,
Here was a Man.
Like him I shall not see again.

Dr. James Compton Burnett

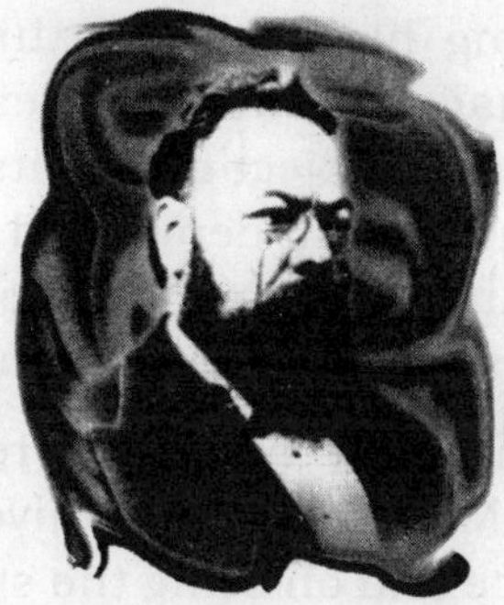

Born : 10-07-1840 Died : 02-04-1901

ANCESTORS & FAMILY

He was the descendant of an old Scotch family, a branch of which come to southern part of Scotland. A famous member of this family was Gilbert Burnett (1643-1715), who was the Bishop of Salisbury and a well known author of ecclesiastical history.

The name Compton was added in 1770 when the grandfather of James Burnett married Miss Compton of Hampshire, a lady of great wealth and personality who desired that Compton be added to the family name. There were several children from this marriage and one of them Charles Compton Burnett, a big landowner was married to Sarah Wilson and to them the hero of this writing was born.

BIRTH

James Compton Burnett was born on 10th of July, 1840 at Redlynch, near Salisbury.

CHILDHOOD & EDUCATION

James was a dark-eyed lovely boy who grew rapidly. By the age of 21 years he had attained the size and weight, which was above that of average, and which he maintained for long years. Born and brought up in the country side, he had to depend on his own devices and was more thoughtful than other youngmen of his age.

He had ordinary English education upto 16 years of age and then he was sent to France where he remained for three years. He travelled on the continent for many years studying Philology for which he had great passion and which can be discerned in the vivid literary style of his writings.

Destiny was guiding him to his future profession. He was fluent in German language and went to Vienna to study medicine. Anatomy was his favourite subject and in its study he devoted two years more than the curriculum demanded. His specimens on the subject prepared by him were highly appreciated and many of them were preserved in the pathological Museum of Vienna.

He passed M.B. in 1869 and then return to join Glasgow University and passed M.B. from that University in 1872. He was in some hospital practice and on seing the success of homoeopathy in the treatment of difficult cases, where allopathy was ineffective, he was inclined to homoeopathy. For M.D. the subject of his thesis was *"Specific Therapeutics"* which has a strong homoeopathic bias and was, as expected, rejected without any judgment of its merit. After a year or two, Burnett sent in another thesis and got his M.D. in 1876.

HIS CONVERSION TO HOMOEOPATHY

Dr. Burnett describes his first contact and success with homoeopathy in Reason No. 1, and in Reason No. 2, he described the cure of his own serious malady in his famous *'Fifty Reasons for Being a Homoeopath'*, about which Clarke says, "No better propagandist booklet was ever published."

The publication of this wonderful book was initiated by a provocative remark by a young allopathic doctor who was taking dinner in a patient's house, accused homoeopaths as quacks. Dr. Burnett's prompt reply was not less dramatic. He said, "Precisely, the old story of abuse and slander of the absent, but no reason. Why, I could give fifty reasons for being a homoeopath, that if not singly at least collectively would convince a stone". He was challenged to produce the fifty reasons, which Burnett did and subsequently the book came into existence.

In *Reason* No. 1 he narrates his mental agonies at the death of an orphan child and his other failures and while he was debating whether to continue in medical practice or to go to America and be a farmer. A medical friend persuaded him to study homoeopathy and he read Dr. Richard Hugheas' *Pharmacodynamics* and *Therapeutics*.

He started using homoeopathic medicines in his own sickness

and the treatment of his patients. The results, thus, obtained convinced and converted him completely. His answer to the criticism was simple yet very strong. He wrote, "What you and the world in general may think of it I care not one straw. I speak well of the bridge that carried me over. For my part I make but one demand of medicine, and one only, viz. *That it shall Cure*. The pathy that will cure is the pathy for me. For of your fairest pathy I can but say:

WHAT CARE I HOW FARE SHE BE
IF SHE BE NOT FAIR TO ME?

He started his medical practice in Chester, and then, inspite of a large practice, shifted to Brikenhead.

He was fascinated by many leading homoeopaths of Liverpool and specially by Dr. John. J. Drysdale's practice and he remained his admirer till last.

In 1877, shifted to London and remained there for 23 years and acquired a large, indeed a very large, practice.

HOMOEOPATHIC PRACTICE & ACTIVITIES

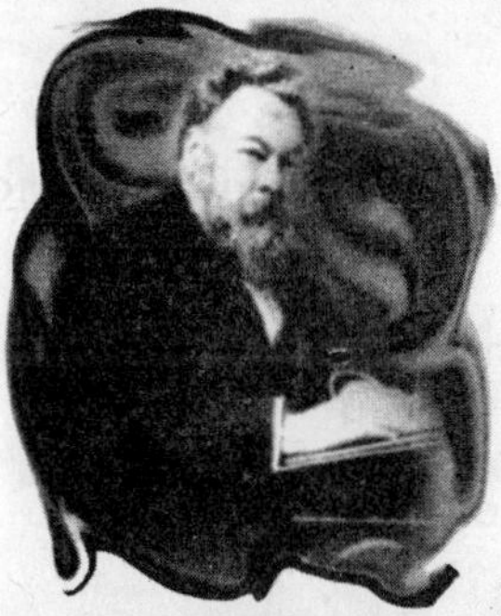

His sincerity, knowledge and devotion to homoeopathy earned him, very soon, a huge practice and recognition by professional brethren. His writings on NATRIUM MURIATICUM and on GOLD AS A REMEDY IN DISEASE were widely read and appreciated.

In 1879 he was chosen to edit THE HOMOEOPATHIC WORLD, a monthly journal of 14 years existence. Dr. Shuldham retired in favour of Dr. Burnett.

In the September 1879 issue of the journal, Dr. Burnett wrote, "For us Homoeopathy means the LAW of SIMILIA in therapeutics. This is the one bond that will bind together.............. . All those who hold that doctrine openly are with us, and we with them. The CRYPTO homoeopaths we despise, the honest haters of homoeopathy we may at least respect. But we cannot respect the mean men who have crawled into professional chairs with the aid of purloined portions of the homoeopathic materia medica and simultaneous abjurations there of. These creeping thing inspire disgust..............".

"............... Unless we omit the word homoeopathy, and also the honourable name of its founder, from our writings, the trade-unionist journals of medicine refuse to print them. Now we will have them WRIT LARGE because of the important truths they symbolize................ homoeopathks may not rest till Homoeopathy is openly taught in all our medical schools, they cannot rest till all disabilities affecting them have been swept away."

He continued as the editor till April 1885 after which Dr. J.H. Clarke took over as the editor of the Journal. It is a often repeated fact that "every writer" is his own best biographer. It will be useful to give in chronological order a complete list of Dr. Burnett's separate works. The works are named in the order in which they were published under the date of their publication, so that it will be easy to follow the progress of the inclination, class, evolution and his services to homoeopathy both as a practitioner and a propagandist of homoeopathy.

LITERARY CONTRIBUTIONS

1879-1895	:	Editor, The Homoeopathic world.
1878	:	Natrium Muriaticum; as a Test of the Doctrine of Drug Dynamization
1879	:	Gold as a Remedy in Disease.
1880	:	On the Prevention of Hare-lip, Cleftpalate, and other Congenital Defects.
1880	:	Ecce Medicus, or Hahnemann as a Man and as a Physician and the Lessons of his life.
1880	:	Curability of Cataract with Medicines.
1880	:	Diseases of the Veins.
1882	:	Supersalinity of the Blood; an Accelerator of Senility and Cause of Cataract.
1882	:	Valvular Disease of The Heart.
1886	:	Diseases of The Skin.
1887	:	Diseases of The Spleen.
1888	:	Fifty Reasons for Being a Homoeopath.
1888	:	Fevers and Blood Poisoning, and Their Treatment, with Special Reference to the Use of Pyrogenium.
1888	:	Tumours of the Breast and their Cure.

1889	:	Neuralgia : Its Causes and Its Remedies.
1889	:	Cataract : Its Nature and Cure.
1890	:	Five Years' (Later edition, Eight Years') Experience in the Cure of Consumption by its own Virus (Bacillinum).
1890	:	On Fistula, and its Cure by Medicines.
1891	:	Greater Disease of the Liver.
1892	:	Ringworm; Constitutional Nature and Cure.
1892	:	Vaccinosis and its Cure by Thuja with remarks on Homoeoprophylaxis
1893	:	Curability of Tumours.
1895	:	Gout and its Cure.
1895	:	Delicate, Backward, Puny and Stunted Children.
1896	:	Organ Diseases of Women.
1898	:	Change of Life in Women.
1901	:	Enlarged Tonsils Cured by Medicines.

It may be mentioned that No. 5 of the above list, "Ecce Medicus" constituted Dr. Burnett's Hahnemann Oration for the year 1880. This was during the active career of the London School of Homoeopathy, Dr. Burnett holding for a brief period the lectureship of Materia Medica in succession to Dr. Hughes.

OTHER CONTRIBUTIONS

This list of Dr. Burnett's books conveys but a partial idea of his literary activity. Not only his own journal, THE HOMOEOPATHIC WORLD, but the British Journal of Homoeopathy and other homoeopathic journals also contain many of his writings.

He introduced the remedy *Bacillinum*, along with other nosodes. He was an intrepid prover, as his proving of *Condurango*, (British Journal of Homoeopathy, July, 1875) alone would suffice to show. But Burnett made provings of many other remedies. Some of these he published, and some have never yet seen the light. He proved the nosode of tubercle, as is mentioned in his cure of consumption. But he proved the viruses of other diseases also, and these he would have published if his life had been prolonged.

He was the one to speak of the concept of "Vaccinosis", that a vaccine could trigger illness. He outlined this in his book, *Vaccinosis*, in 1884.

THE DEMISE

His engagements prevented any physical exercise but although he was always playful in disposition there were unmistakable signs of the approaching end. In the last part of his life he was unusually deliberate in going upstairs. The night before he died, some of his patients observed that his hands were icy-cold which was very unusual because in the coldest weather his hands used to remain warm. In the night of April 1st, 1901, he dined as usual at his hotel, Holborn Viaduc Hotel, and retired as usual to his room. It was only in the morning, when his breakfast and carriage were kept waiting that the sad discovery was made that he must have passed away just as he was retiring to rest. Dr. Burnett used to say "My only hope is that I may die in harness" which seems to have been fulfilled.

The death of a brother about a fortnight before his own seems to have affected him deeply and could be the reason why a fortnight before his death he made a new will.

Dr. Clarke says, "The holiday he had denied himself so long had come at last.......... . The great heart had worn itself out."

The OBITUARY in the famous DAILY TIMES of April, 5th, 1901 said, "the force of his personality was felt by all who came in contact with him and his patients were attached to him in a more than ordinary degree .... For many years he had taken no holiday longer than five days at a time, and it is probably to this excessive strain that the sudden failure of his powers is due. The cause of death was disease of the heart. He leaves a widow and family."

Another famous news paper WEST MINSTOR GAZETTE wrote on 4th April, "Many will regret to hear the death of Dr. Burnett of 86, Wimpole Street and 2, Finsbury Cirus...... . For many years he has carried on one of the largest consulting practices in London .... He was the greatest living exponent of the Paracelsic doctrine of Organopathy."

HOMOEOPATHIC HEROES OF BURNETT

Dr. John J. Drysdale, M.D.

Burnett in the dedication of the second American addition of his CURABILITY OF TUMOURS BY MEDICINES wrote "the memory of the father of scientific homoeopathy in great Britan, John J. Drysdale, this little volume is dedicated in affection, admiration and gratitude." Clarke wrote, "It may fairly be said that John Drysdale was Burnett's chief here among his contemporaries."

Dr. Alfred E. Hawkes of liverpool

Burnett dedicated his FIFTY REASONS OF BEING A HOMOEOPATH to Hawkes "for having induced him to put the homoeopthy of Hahnemann to the test in bed side experience ...." Although Dr. Drysdale was highest in the esteem of Burnett but it was Alfred E. Hawkes who introduced him to homoeopathy.

Rademacher

Burnett dedicated his GREATER DISEASES OF THE LIVER to Rademacher whom he called — "The Resuscitator of PARACELSIC ORGANOPATHY". He has praised Rademacher in his "Diseases of the Spleen" also.

Henry Goullon

Burnett dedicated his TUMOURS OF THE BREAST (published in 1888) to Henry Goullon, M.D. of Weimar, Germany.

Paracelsus

Burnett regarded Paracelsus as a forerunner of Hahnemann. About Burnett's admiration for Paracelsus, Clarke Wrote, "Burnett's admiration for Paracelsus will be in constant evidence .... He ranks second only to Hahnemann himself in Burnett's Calendar of Medical Heroes".

Dr. William Earnest Boyd

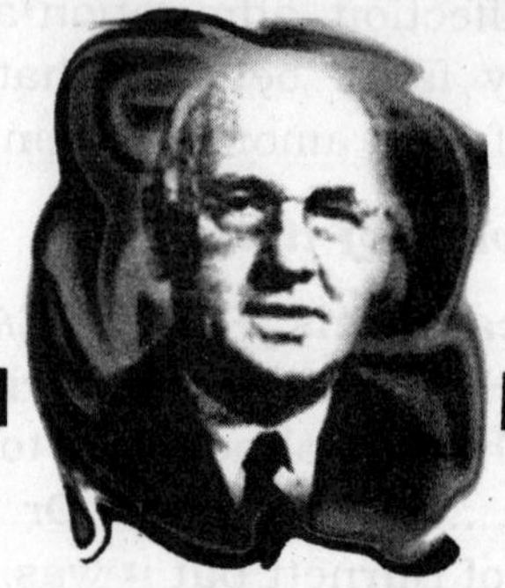

Born : 21-05-1891 **Died : 1955**

Dr. Boyd, was born on May 21, 1891 in Glasgow. He was educated at the Glasgow Acedemy and the Glasgow University, from where he took the M.A., M.B., Ch. B. and M.D. degrees. During the World War-I, he sarved as a Surgeon in the Royal Navy. Later he joined the Homoeopathic Faculty in 1919. It was due to the influence of Dr. Gibson Miller that he owed his initial knowledge and interest in Homoeopathy. From 1920 onwards, he was Physician and Radiologist to the Glasgow Homoeopathic Hospital. He was the founder and first Director of the Boyd Medical Research Trust Labotatories. He was member of numerous learned societies, such as the Faraday, Society Glasgow; the Royal philosophical society, Glasgow; the Society of Physical Medicine branch of the British Medical Association; the Institute of Radiology and the British Institute of Engineers. He was a fellow of the Royal Society of Medicine, the Institute of Electronics and a Member of the Faculty of Homoeopathy.

Between 1922 and August 1954, be contributed many papers on homoeopathic or bio-chemical research to the British Homoeopathic Journal. In 1936 he published a monograph entitled 'Low Potencies of Homoeopathy'. Dr. Boyd proved by the experiments on his Emanometer beyond any shadow of doubt that the presence of a power exists in 30th potency of *Mercuric Chloride*. He thus vindicated the clinical insight of Hahnemann, who could not explain how such an inconceivably diluted solution as the 30th potency, lacking even a single molicule of the original drug, could cure the sick person.

Dr. Hahnemann used the terms *'Spiritual Vital Force'* and later *'Dynamis'* to explain the phenomenon of cure based on the Law of

Similars. The bio-physical or the dynamic state of the sick person should be similar to the dynamic influence produced by the drug on a healthy prove to neutralise the vital disorder. Ofcourse, the Law of Similars as enunciated by Hahnemann belonged to the biological sphere, and therefore, could not satisfy the scientific minds who think in terms of physics and chemistry. It was Dr. Boyd who cam forward to prove by experimental verifications that who power released by drug is a kind of emanations which could he measured and applied.

Earlier, George Starr, Abrahm, Stearns and others in U.S.A. were on this tract. They found that a homoeopathic remedy has palpable effects on the sick persons. The eye reflex and percussion notes, and pulse show definite effects of the homoeopathic remedy. Dr. W. R. Mc Crac has shown by means of his electrophysical tests that a group remedy could be found which leads to the selection of the correct homoeopathic remedy. Dr. Boericke has shown by his flocculation test that the emanations of the sick person are similar to the emanations of the correct homoeopathic remedy.

Dr. Boyd discovered that there are some sort of emanations produced by homoeopathically prepared drugs which act only on the tissues to which each individual drug is fitted and only on the folks to whom it is tuned. There is evidence of a kind suggesting that disorganisation of healthy state of body is due to effects on people or emanations from substance they take or sources to which they are exposed. If this is so, what a vista is opened out for fine methods of diseases! This discovery of 'Divining Methods': flocculation tests, electro-physical tests and radiosthesia are latest devices for further advancement of Homoeopathy to prevent and cure innumerable acute and chronic diseases mildly, quickly and permanently. Then only the mission of Hahnemann shall be fulfilled.

Dr. Hem Chandra Bysack

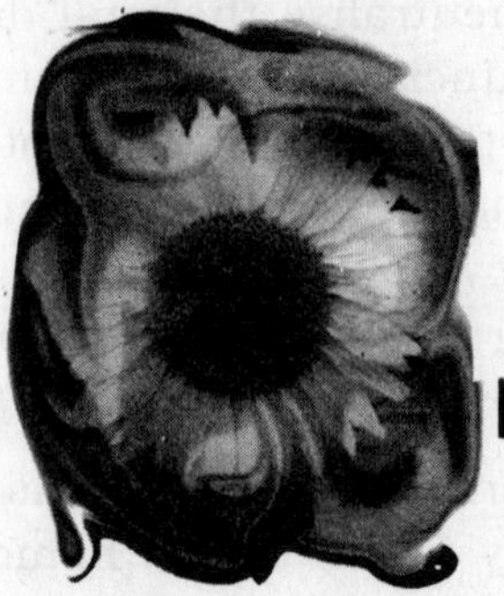

Died : 1963

Dr. Hem Chandra Bysack was a staunch Hahnemannion homoeopathic physician practicing at his house in the Gheewalon Ka Rasta, Raipur. Neither he stoop down to profit, nor he yield to the slackening of strict diet regimen. So he did not attract a crowd of clientele, but adhered to the principles of homoeopathy. He practiced from 1941 until his untimely death in November 1963.

Section-B : Dr. Bysack, Hem Chandra

SECTION-C .... Page 47 to 65

C-1 ***Dr. Caspari, Carl***
(Born: 1798 / Died: 15-02-1828) 48

C-2 ***Dr. Chand, Diwan***
(Born: 03-08-1887 / Died: 14-05-1961) 52

C-3 ***Dr. Chatterjee, D.N.***
(Born: 1903 / Died: 1961) 59

C-4 ***Dr. Chowdhury, Bankim***
(Born: 1904 / Died: 1977) 60

C-5 ***Dr. Clarke, John Henry***
(Born: 1853 / Died: 24-11-1931) 62

C-6 ***Dr. Close, Stuart M.***
(Born: 14-11-1860 / Died: 26-05-1929) 65

Dr. Carl Caspari

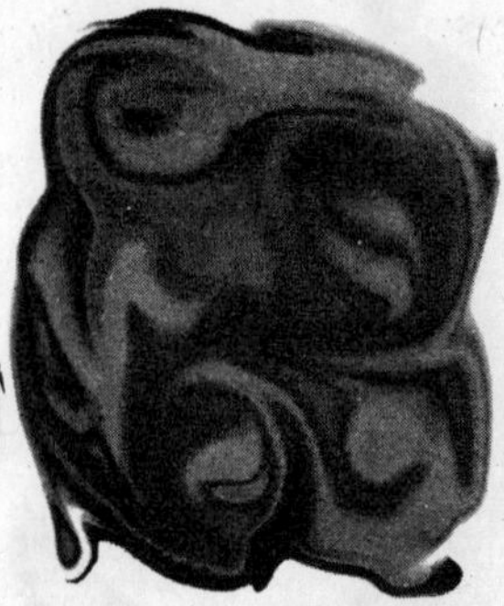

Born : 1798 **Died : 15-02-1828**

SOURCE MATERIALS

1. Dr. T.L. Bradford: The Pioneers of Homoeopathy, P. 10.
2. Rapou : Histoire de la Doctrine Medicale Homoeopathique, P. 130-36, 208.
3. Kleinert : Geschichte der Homoeopathie, P. 130.
4. Homoeopathic World, Vol. XXIV, P. 497.
5. Allg. Homoeopathische Zeitung, Vol. XXXIX, P. 289.
6. North West Journal of Homoeopathy, Vol. IV, P. 233.

BIRTH & EARLY LIFE

Carl Caspari was the son of a village priest and the grandson of Prof. D. Scnott of Eschorlau, near Delitzsch. He graduated from Leipzig.

EDUCATION & ACHIEVEMENTS

He delivered a course of lectures on practical surgery to the students of Leipzig. He was fascinated by homoeopathy and relinquished a bright and lucrative future easily accessible to him in any famous school of surgery. He published "My Observations Upon Homoeopathy". Since he had excellent relations with the important physicians of allopathy as well as homoeopathy, he attempted to reconcile the two doctrines and tried to propagate an amalgamation between the two system. But during the later part of his life, he left this idea and became a zealous homoeopath. He was convinced of the irrationality of allopathy and was of opinion that with the help of homoeopathic medicines surgical diseases can be

---

Section-C : Dr. Caspari, Carl

treated successfully. He was offered the Chair of homoeopathy at the University of Cracow, but refused it to continue his researches. He excelled in didactic writings. His primary interest was in surgery and did some research work on the scope of homoeopathy and allopathy in surgical diseases and established that homoeopathy has greater applicability in so-called surgical diseases.

According to Rapou, Caspari made a special study of electricity in connection with homoeopathic therapeutics and spoke highly of the healing powers of electricity.

It is said that Hahnemann did not like him because of his suggestion and attempt to amalgamate allopathy and homoeopathy.

Hartmann wrote about Caspari, "At this time (1826) two men were living whose premature death was a sad loss to homoeopathy, for both were gifted men and their works testify their powers of mind such as the creator enstrusts to but few. I refer to Dr. Caspari and Dr. Hartlaub Sr."

Hartmann describes Caspari's characters as "not quite accessible by every one" and "possessed of an insufferable haughtiness which seemed to be based upon a fancy that he was exalted above all others".

Caspari accomplished much at the time when homoeopathy needed perfection in every direction. He comprehend his subjects completely and enriched the science by its development.

He understood that the rapid spread of homoeopathy depends on the sympathy of the public and he tired to achieve this by his popular book, *"Homoeopathic Domestic Medicine"* .

In the beginning of 1828 he was attacked with small-pox during an epidemic and became delirious and shot himself through his head on 15th of February, 1828, at the young age of about 30 years.

CONTRIBUTIONS

Caspari was the first person to write a book on homoeopathic pharmacy. He proved *Carbo vegetabilis* before Hahnemann. He was the first to take the study of Electricity as a therapeutic agent.

His *"My Experience in Homoeopathy : an Unprejudiced Estimation of Hannemann's System"* was published in 1823.

Hartmann observed, "And who knows whether by his proving

of CARBO VEGETABILIS he might not have excited Hahnemann to undertake the proving of both the charcoals. I am not quite positive as regards this last fact, but remember that Hahnemann was at one time quite angry at Caspari and cannot tell whether it was because he was always displeased with those who anticipated him."

Caspari was a man of intellect and great attainments, and would have rendered homoeopathy many an essential service.

HOMOEOPATHIC WRITINGS

1823 : My Experience in Homoeopathy : An Unprejudiced Estimation of Hahnemann's System, Leipzig, Lehnhold.

1825 : Handbook of Dietetics for all Ranks, arranged according to the Homoeopathic principles, Leipzig, Lehnhold.

1825 : Homoeopathic Dispensatory for Physicians and Druggists. Edited by Hartmann, Leipzig, Baumgartner. Fifth edition, 1834; Seventh edition, 1852. It was also published under the title: Homoeopathic Pharmacopoeai.

1825 : Catechism of Homoeopathic Dietetics for the Sick, Leipzig, Baumgartner. Second edition, edited by Dr. Gross, Leipzig, 1831, later published under the title: Catechism for the Sick.

1826 : Homoeopathic Domestic and Traveller's Physician. Edited by Fr. Hartmann, Leipsic, Baumgartner. Fifth edition, 1835, Tenth edition, 1851, (was also translated into English).

1828 : Demonstration of the Truth of the Homoeopatic Method of Healing as founded on the Laws of Nature, According to the experience of Bigel, Leipzig, Baumgartner.

1829 : Dispensatorium Homoeopathicum, Edited by Hartmann, Leipzig, Baumgartner (Latin).

1834 : Homoeopathic Pathology; also under the title Library for Homoeopathic Medicine and Materia Medica, Leipsic, Focke. 1827-28. Second edition, 1834.

Volume 1. Homoeopathic Pathology; Volume II. General Homoeopathic Diagnosis; Volume III. General Homoeopathic Therapeutics.

OTHER WRITINGS

1822 : De Jejunii in Morbis Sanandis Usu, Leipzig, Rueckmann.

1821 : Anatomico-chirurgical Treatise on Dislocations together with a postcript on complicated dislocations, Leipzig, Kohler.

1823 : Medical House Friend, or Self-help in the Treatment of Diseases, Leipzig, Leich.

1823 : Injuries to the Head and their Treatment, from the oldest times to the present, with new ideas and A Treatise on Inflammation, Leipzig, Lehnhold.

1823 : Stone in the Kidney, Bladder and Gall-bladder; its origin and chemical diagnostic and therapeutic consideration, Leipzig, Fleischer.

1823 : Vade Macum of Spring-Curing, or a Treatise on the Judicious Use of Herbs and Bath-cures, etc., Leipzig, Lehnhold.

1824 : System of Surgical Dressings Systematically Arranged and Reduced to a Science, Leipzig, Zirges, First edition, 1822.

1825 : Catechism of the Manner of Living for Young Wives, Leipzig, Baumgartner.

1826 : Investigation as to the Medical Virtues of Charcoal from Beech-wood, Leipzig, Baumgartner.

1834 : Hand-Book of the Newly Married, Leipzig, Baumgartner, 1825. Second edition was edited by Hartmann.

Dr. Diwan Jai Chand

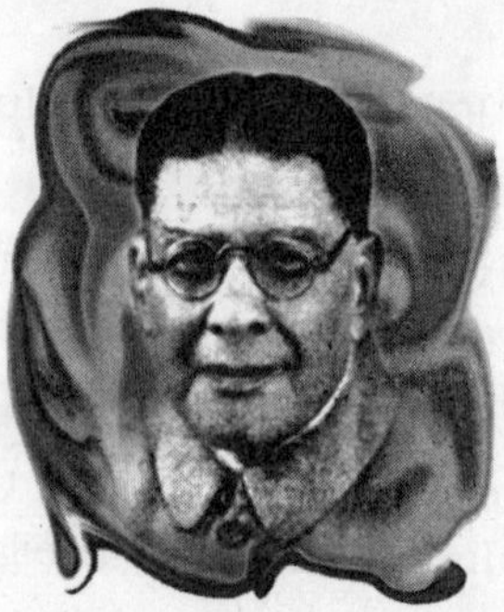

Born : 03-08-1887

Died : 14-05-1961

"Dr. Diwan Jai Chand is Homoeopathy and Homoeopathy is Dr. Diwan Jai Chand. Go and meet him." This is what a young Homoeopath was told when he was going to visit Lahore in the thirties. This Dr. Diwan Jai Chand, whose name has been a byword for Homoeopathy and who is held as the Father of Homoeopathy in Northern India, passed away on the 14th of May, 1961 mourned not only by his family and friends, but by the entire Homoeopathic fraternity and the tens of thousands that derived benefit from his treatment.

Born on 3rd July, 1887 at Rahim Yar Khan in Bhawalpur State (now in West Pakistan) he had his education upto High School there. He passed his Intermediate from D.A.V. College, Lahore. One of his subjects was Philosophy. This helped him later in life to critically examine the soundness of Hahnemann's principles of Homoeopathy. He had his initial medical education at the K.E. Medical College, Lahore. He left for U.K. in 1910 and returned in 1913 after passing L.R.C.P., L.R.C.S. (Edin), L.R.F.P. & S. (Glas.), D.P.H. (Edin), D.T.M. (L'Pool), L.M. (Dub.) and doing an apprenticeship in Bacteriology and Public Health work. He had a brilliant academic career and was a scholarship holder all through. During his stay at the K.E. Medical College, Lahore, he was the first recipient of the Beli Ram Lamont Medal in Anatomy and secured certificates of honour in Medicine and Ophthalmic Surgery besides some other subjects. He passed with great distinction all his examinations in the Medical College, Lahore as also in U.K. and Ireland.

The certificates that he received from his professors in U.K. speak with forceful eloquence of his exceptional abilities such as, "Exceptionally skilful and painstaking and most enthusiastic of my students... At the D.P.H. Examination made a particularly brilliant appearance... His study of Public Health has been exceptionally through... I know of no one who has better fitted himself to undertaking Public Health work in the East..." and so on. His memory was so remarkable that he could reproduce pages verbatum and give references of pages from memory. At an Examination in Physiology, he requested that he be given a seat in the front row right under the nose of the invigilator as he offered to reproduce the class notes of the professor (Prof. Caleb) word by word and did not wish to be under any suspicion of copying. At Edinburgh once the Prof. of Public Health was having difficulty in searching for a certain Public Health Act in the Book, of which he was the author, Dr. Diwan Jai Chand told him the page on which it was given and could also reproduce it verbatum. This prodigal memory was his great asset right till the end. As a matter of fact, during the last two years of his life when his sight was gradually failing, and he could not read much, his memory got even more acute and he could always guide other doctors where to look for a particular information and in which part of the page.

His great reverence for his teachers was of the classical type. After acquiring all the qualifications he was going to take Examination for the coveted Indian Medical Service and had sent in his application and completed all formalities when perchance he met his professor in the street. On learning of his plans the professor told him, "Dr. Jai Chand! I am shocked. A person of austere habits like you, who is a vegetarian, a tea-totaller and of such rare brilliance and diligence should not rot his life in the I.M.S. Instead I can offer you a research post is Bacteriology and Public Health and would consider it a privilege if you work with me or else I can have you sent for such work to British Africa, that would be more becoming for your talents." On receiving this advice he immediately gave up the idea of joining Indian Medical Service and returned his rail ticket. However, he declined the rare honour of offer of research post there because of family considerations and to return to his motherland.

On return from U.K. he joined service with the Punjab Government as Deputy Sanitary Commissioner in the Public Health Department. He was one of the first Indians to be appointed to that high post. He resigned soon after due to his independent nature and nationalist political leanings. He than started his Clinic at Lahore in 1915, probably one of the first exclusively consulting physician. He was the Secretary of Lahore Medical Union (Allopathic

Body), the precursor of the Punjab Branch of Indian Medical Association.

His introduction and conversion to Homoeopathy was just an accident, for initially in common with his Allopathic colleagues he was very bigoted and a denouncer of Homoeopathy, of which, of course, he knew nothing. It was in the cause of national political movement that he came to reluctantly teach Midwifery and Gynecology at a Homoeopathic College. A casual perusal of some books at the college library in the few spare moments before his lecture, interested him in the science. A further study convinced him of the scientific nature of Homoeopathy and the clinical trails were very gratifying, sometimes bordering on magical. Once he was thoroughly convinced he decided to practise this system ridiculed by his colleagues. All the medicines in his dispensary he threw into a gutter near his clinic rather than sell them to somebody. When questioned about it he said, "I cannot sell poison, what is not good for my patients is not good for other doctor's patients also". People called him mad and he had to suffer ridicule and financial and social privations because till then no qualified doctor had taken to the practice of Homoeopathy in Northern India. But he stood steadfast in his belief and when he started to cure those declared incurable by the Allopaths he regained public esteem and gradually his fame spread far and wide.

As a physician he was remarkable and such was the efficacy of the treatment administered by him that he dominated the profession for three decades in the prepartition Punjab and later in Delhi and came to be known as "a great healer", "a miracle man" and "a Messiah" who could revive those that are nearly dead.

He made himself available to all sections of society and his very extensive practice ranged from the humblest to the highest in the Land. He had among his clients people like Pt. Moti Lal Nehru (a great patron of Homoeopathy), Sir Sunder Singh Majithia, Sir Shahabudin, Bhai Vir Singh, Sir Abdul Qadir and his family, Bawa Sawan Singh of Beas, Maulana Abul Kalam Azad and many Central Government Ministers, the Maharajas and the nobility. Majority of Europeans and Anglo-Indians of Lahore were his patients. He used to be called to see patients as far away as Karachi and Calcutta and of course all over Northern India, and used to send medicines to patients even in Africa, Burma, Far East and sometimes U.K. The success of his practice can be gauged from the fact that among the doctors (including Allopaths) at Lahore he paid the highest Income

Tax. He was thus instrumental in raising the dignity and status of Homoeopathy.

For some time he was the President of the Punjab Homoeopathic League at Lahore. He was the founder and Principal of National Homoeopathic College in Lahore in the early twenties but had to close it down after some years for want of enough trained personnel to man it. After independence of the country in 1947, he had to shift to Delhi as a refugee from West Pakistan and establish his Clinic in New Delhi. He was President of the All India Institute of Homoeopathy, Delhi Branch, for some years. Later he mostly remained aloof from different associations so as to effectively mediate and bring about unity. He enjoyed the confidence of all sections and was ever ready to espouse and help the Homoeopathic cause in which at every quarter his help was needed.

At Lahore for 30 years till the time of partition he conducted a pharmacy, the National Homoeopathic Pharmacy, to be able to provide books, genuine medicines and other sundries to the numerous people he converted to Homoeopathy in Punjab as propagation of Homoeopathy became a life mission. He also founded and edited an excellent journal, "Health and Homoeopathy". For paucity of enough material of the requisite standard it became almost a single handed effort and so had to be discontinued after some time.

He served on the Punjab Homoeopathic Enquiry Committee before partition of the country. In 1996, he led a deputation to the Health Minister in the Interim National Government and his sound arguments and enthusiastic approach made a very favourable impression and the deputation was promised that steps would be taken to recognize Homoeopathy. In 1948, he was appointed a Member of the Homoeopathic Enquiry Committee and he put in lot of labour in producing convincing material for the Allopath Members of the Committee and for final incorporation in the report and making it favourable to Homoeopathy. In 1952, he was appointed a Member of the Ad Hoc Committee on Homoeopathy. In 1956, this was changed to the Homoeopathic Advisory Committee of the Ministry of Health, Government of India, and he continued to be a Member there till his death taking an active part in its deliberations and always trying to establish Homoeopathy on a firm footing and securing for it equal status with Allopathy. He also served on the Research and Technical Sub. Committee of the Homoeopathic Advisory Committee. In 1956, he was again a member of the

Indigenous and Homoeopathy System Committee of the Planning Commission. Besides that he had the distinction of being the only Homoeopath appointed to the Health Programmes Panel of the Planning Commission. He was thus a member of every committee on Homoeopathy and a senior guide.

He was an entirely self-made man. To go abroad for studies he raised the money by selling his wife's jewellery and raising loans. He was sincere, honest and truthful to the core and he always maintained that honesty and truth increase life by keeping a person at peace with his conscience and thus fearless in facing the world.

A non-professional activity of note was the tremendous labour Dr. Jai Chand put in as the Chairman of Peoples Bank of Northern India Ltd., to try and save this premier bank of the Punjab from going into liquidation and thus save from ruin countless families. It is highly creditable that it was all a labour of love as his work, done at great professional and personal sacrifices, was all honorary though it could have fetched him many lacs of rupees. Seeing his banking abilities and sincerity in work he was offered a post in another bank which carried a salary double than his income. He rejected it outright without a second thought with the remark, "the pleasure I get in curing the sick and suffering people cannot be compensated by any amount of money."

He was a philanthropist and particularly for the cause of Homoeopathy he always opened his purse wide. At Lahore he contributed to a Homoeopathic Association Rs. 150/- per month to run a Homoeopathic Charitable Dispensary. After the partition of Punjab, in spite of the heavy losses sustained in that political holocaust, he made a provision of Rs. 40,000 for a Homoeopathic Hospital, even though it was difficult for him to Spare that sum. Out of this he made a handsome contribution towards the construction of a Hospital by the Roshan Lal Trust Society at Meerut (U.P.). He had been the Chairman of this Trust for nearly 30 years. He was a publicity shy man and never published what he considered to be meagre contributions. He used to say that, "My contribution to Homoeopathy is that I have put both my sons in its service." At Lahore he was once approached by his Allopathic colleagues to donate for a College. He offered to give Rs. 50,000 if they provided a chair for Homoeopathy there.

He was a rebel by nature who will never compromise with wrong and standby his convictions even if it meant sacrifice and suffering. He prized the approval of his conscience more than the routine ways of the multitude and never attempted to float with the tide of popular opinion, but was ever firm and steadfast in his devotion to what he believed to be true and right. At the tender age of four years he left his parental home to go and live with his grandfather as he felt he had been thrashed without any reason. From his childhood he had a passion for medicine and at the age of 17 years he struck to his resolve to study medicine and suffer all the privations of losing financial assistance and being disinherited by his family for they wanted him to join service and fixed up the coveted job of a Naib Tehsildar. He actually lived very thriftily and supported himself by scholarship till the family compromised and permitted his medical education. Later in life when he was convinced of the scientific nature and superiority of Homoeopathy he took its practice in spite of all the ridicule, social and professional boycott and initial financial loss. Politically his rebellious nature against the British rulers was shown by his active participation in the Congress movement. For some time he was the President of the Lahore Branch. He was a habitual wearer of Khadi exclusively since the very inception of the Khadi movement when he burnt all his foreign clothes in the bonfire. To promote the use of Swadeshi goods he financed a shop and that meant a sacrifice of Rs. 45,000. In the religious and social sphere he as a free thinker and of advanced views and regardless of public opinion he preached against many harmful though aged honoured practices as caste system. He was a member of the Jat Pat Torak Mandal, a staunch prohibitionist and puritan in outlook. In 1917 he became a member of Theosophical Society and Universal Brotherhood of Mme Annie Besant. He was not demonstrative in his religion but religious in his living. And what he preached he practised. He encouraged and brought about intercaste marriages in the family and simplified all the ceremonies. He was too simple to be ostentatious, too great to stoop to vain display. He was a true *karma-yogi,* and would continue his work unruffled even in the face of emotional upheavals and such personal tragedies as the death of his closest kith and kin.

Dr. Jai Chand was an extremely hard working person and tireless in his energy. From the early age of 13 years he developed the habit of getting up at 2 A.M. and devoting the whole of the latter part of the night for studies. The habit continued almost till the end. He was a voracious reader and except for the few sleeping hours one would always find him reading a magazine, journal or book. This was so even when he went for a walk or while he took his food, his interest being more in reading than in eating and he hardly ever recalled what he had eaten. His interests were very wide and one could see him reading on all sorts of subjects. Work was his worship. After an attack of Coronary Thrombosis in 1956 whenever it was suggested that he work less and take more rest he would say that there is a long rest ahead and it could not be far in the indifferent state of his health so let him earn that rest. His associates used to joke with him that he worked 366 days in a leap year for he never observed even a half holiday on Sundays. It was fairly normal for him to see patients almost continuously for 12-14 hours as he did not take any lunch. The only holiday he had in his life was in 1926 and he spent it mostly in reading books. Even when his last illness forced him to retirement he would lecture animatedly for long hours to some doctors who used to gather around him. He was a perfectionist by habit and did nothing half heartedly. Whatever he undertook he did with great zeal. In keeping with his literary taste he had one of the world's best library of Homoeopathic books.

With his passing away the Homoeopathic profession has lost one of its best and most experienced exponents. Rarely can it be said of any human being that no one can fill his place, but of Dr. Jai Chand, it is as true as ever it can be. The blow sustained by the Homoeopathic profession in his death is inexpressible and simply irrepairable. To most of the Homoeopaths he was a true guide, philosopher and friend — one who could enter into their difficulties and from whom they received much encouragement — he was a real haven of refuge. His life of simple living and high thinking and the ideas he set himself will always remain as a beacon light of inspiration and source of courage in the storms that come in the way of progress of Homoeopathy and a glorious example to follow.

In the words of a poet —

"He is not dead whose glorious mind lifts thine on high
To live in hearts, we have behind, is not to die."

Dr. D.N. Chatterjee

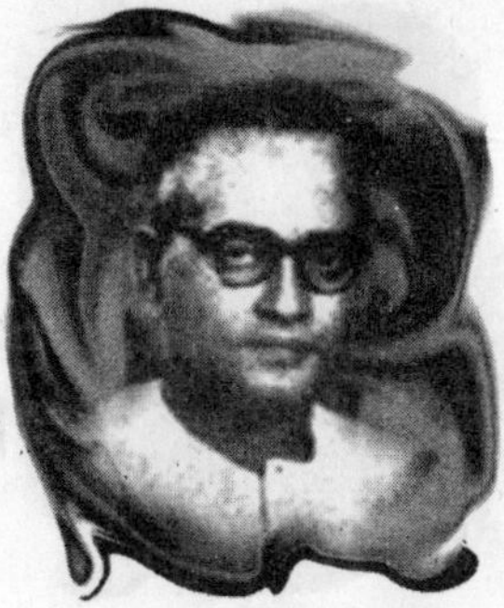

Born : 1903 Died : 1961

Dr. D. N. Chatterjee was born in 1903 at Bejagaon in Vikrampore now in Bangladesh. He graduated from the Bengal Allen Homoeopathic Medical College. He then became a Professor in the D. N. De Homoeopathic College. In 1927, he founded a phgarmacy the 'Bengal Homoeo Stores'. In 1928 he started the publication of a homeopathic journal, titled 'Homoeopathic Bulletin'.

He wrote a number of books amongst which may be mentioned: Family Physician, Drugs of India, Biochemistry, treatment of Female Diseases, etc. He was for some time the Vice-President of the Indian Homoeopathic Medical Association and International Hahnemannian Society of India. He was the member of the Executive Committee of the State Homoeopathic Faculty, and the Principal of D. N. De Homoeopathic Medical College and Hospital (Formerly Dunham College). He passed away on Nov. 29, 1961.

Dr. Bankim Chowdhury

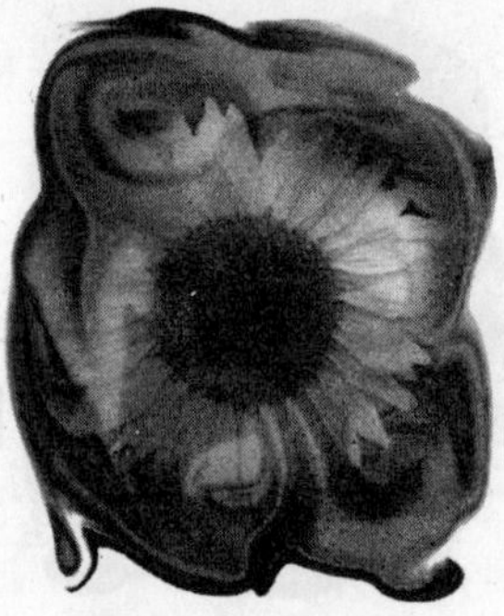

Born : 1904 **Died : 1977**

Dr. Bankim Choudhury, founder of Midnapore Homoeopathic Medical College and Hospital and Kharagpore Homoeopathic Medical College and Hospital and torchbearer of homoeopathic science in Midnapore District, was born at Jhantla, in the District of Midnapore on June 9, 1904. He had his academic education in Hindu School, on completion of which he went to Bankura to study allopathic medical science at Bankura Sammilani Medical College and Hospital. He was conferred L.M.F. in 1928 from that institution. During his studies he used to enjoy scholarship from Midnapore District Board. Dr. Chowdhuri was successful in his medical profession; still he forsook allopathic practice in the interest of finding out more truth in Homoeopathy. The miraculous effect of one dose of Solidago-virga given to his dying father during his urinary trouble, absolutely converted him into a homoeopath.

Thus Dr. Chowdhuri came out successful with flying colours in homoeopathic science from state faculty of homoeopathic science from State Faculty of Homoeopathic Medicine, West Bengal in the year 1944, as a D.M.S.

Soon after that he opened a Charitable Homoeopathic Dispensary in the Midnapore town. To this he added a College of Homoeopathic Medicine, which was followed by a Hospital Medicine, which was followed by a Hospital at the same place. He was conferred Honorary M.D. by the Council of Homoeopathic Medicine, West Bengal in recognition of his valiant fight and sacrifice for Homoeopathy in 1975. He founded Kharapore Homoeopathic Medical College and Hospital at the fag end of his life along with several health centres in the rural areas. He held

Section-C : Dr. Chowdhury, Bankim

the membership of the Council of Homoepathic Medicine, West Bengal since its inception till his demise.

Death came to him with silent foot-steps and he faced the fate with a smiling countenance on the April 5, 1977, but his yeoman service to the homoeopathic science will live for ever and speak of his glory to poterity for ages to come.

Dr. John Henry Clarke

Born : 1853

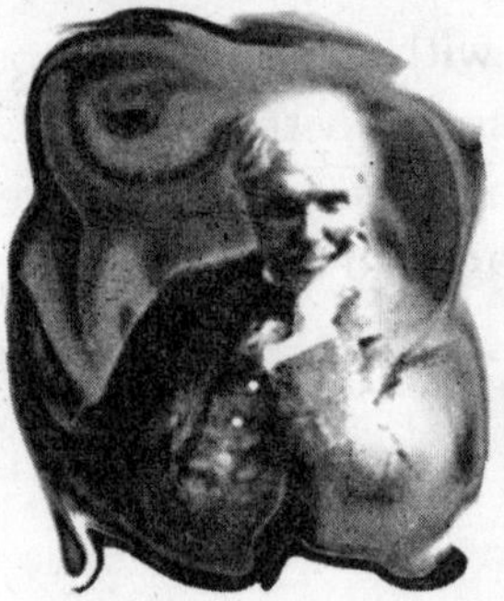

Died : 24-11-1931

John Henry Clarke, M.D., was one of the student of Richard Hughes. Educated at Edinburgh he received his degree in 1877.

He was opposed by many Homoeopaths after he began to associate with *high potency* prescribers in Liverpool like Thomas Skinner, and Edward Berridge.

From 1885 to 1898 and again from 1923 until his death, Clarke worked as an editor for the *Homoeopathic World*.

Dr. Edgar Whittaker says of Clarke, in Homoeopathic World, January 1932, "Clarke described the other leading members of the cooper club as 'the three most potent influences on the evolution of British Homoeopathy today', and wrote in 1901 : "It is not too much to say that during the last twenty years Burnett has been the most powerful, the most fruitful, the most original force in homoeopathy'. Clarke was himself a physician to be reckoned with, and in time the another of a medical encylopedia which rivaled Hughes."

Clarke was a prolific writer. He used to visit his patients in a horse-drawn carriage which was like an office inside, complete with a writing desk, as Clarke was found of writing he never lost an opportunity to work on his books.

Margaret Tyler said: "A brilliant writer, Clarke wielded a very caustic pen. But his influence for good might have been greater had he been less fierce, and made a little allowance for those whose real sin was ignorance. The old school was to be bullied and rated. Ignorance was 'cussedness' to be bludgeoned into knowledge — rather than tactfully helped and taught. He was so sure on his own ground, that he had no mercy on the man on the other side of the fence. 'Pandering to the allopaths' was his name for courtesy to men who are, after all, our brethren in the healing art. He set his fly-traps with vinegar."

Clarke supported the lay movement in homoeopathy. He believed that it did not matter if the remedy is prescribed by a qualified prescriber or not. He wrote many books for the untrained worker and domestic prescriber.

Clarke established his own publishing house for his books — The Homoeopathic Publishing Company — because no reputable publishing house wanted to publish his work. Clarke's literary work include the following.

1885 — The Prescriber, 9th Editions.

1886 — Revolution in Medicine.

1887— Odium Medicine and Homoeopathy : The Times Correspondence.

1888 — Indigestion : Its causes and Cure.

1890 — Dictionary of Domestic Medicine.

1893 — Cholera Diarrhea and Dysentery.

1893 — Therapeutics of Serpent Poisons.

1894 — Homoeopathy : All about it.

1895 — Diseases of the Heart and Arteries.

1899 — Catarrh Colds and Grippe.

1900 — Dictionary of Practical Materia Medica, Three volumes.

1904 — Clinical Repertory.

1904 — Rheumatism and Sciatica.

1904 — Life and works of James Compton Burnett.

1905 — Homoeopathy Explained.

1907 — Thomas Skinner : A Biographical Sketch.

1908 — Radium as an Internal Remedy.

1908 — The Cure of Tumors by Medicine.

1915 — Gunpowder as a War Remedy.

1923 — Hahnemann & Paracelsus.

1931 — Dr. Skinner's Grand Characteristics.

Constitutional Medicine.

Foundations of Materia Medica.

Non-Surgical Diseases of the Glands.

Apart from homoeopathy, Clarke wrote on other subjects also. He wrote many anti-Jewish and anti-German tracts. He was an outspoken anti-nivisectionist. Clarke served as a treasurer and Vice-president of a group known as "Britons", who later became the British Union of Fascists. During this time he wrote five books: The Call of the Sword (1917); England under the Heel of the Jew (1918); Democracy and Shylocracy; White Labour versus Red (1922); A Patriotic Fund to Fight the Hidden Hand (1923).

Dr. Stuart M. Close

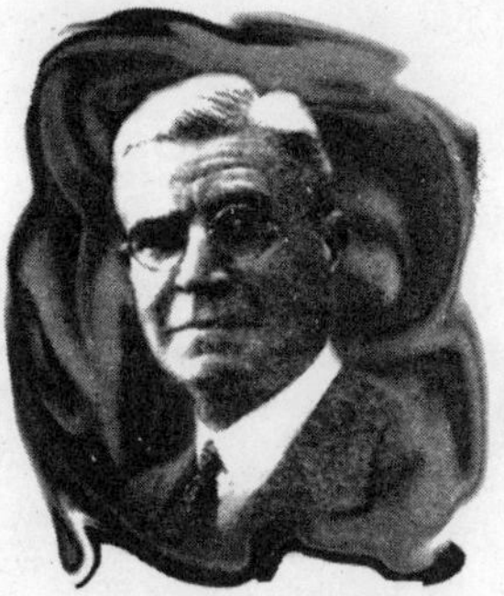

Born : 14-11-1860 **Died : 26-05-1929**

Close, M.D., was born on 24th of November, 1860. Before converting to homoeopathy Close was interested to study law.

When Close was 19 yrs. old his father died, in 1879. After his father's death his mother re-married a homoeopathic physician. Close studied the Organon with his Step-father. He attended the medical school in California for two years and completed his graduation from New York Homoeopathic Medical College, in 1885. Close worked with P.P. Wells and Bernhardt Fincke after finishing the school. He set up his practice in Brooklyn, New York.

Close was the founder of *Brooklyn Homoeopathic Union,* a group devoted to the study of the principles of pure Hahnemannian homoeopathy. He founded this union in the year 1897.

In 1905, Close was elected as the president of the *International Hahnemannian Association.* He was professor of Homoeopathic Philosophy at *New York Homoeopathic Medical College* from 1909 to 1913. Initially his lectures were published in the *Homoeopathic Recorder.* Later, these lectures were complied and published in form of a book, *The Genius of Homoeopathy.* It is one of the most condensed book on homoeopathic philosophy. Close had one of the finest homoeopathic libraries in the country.

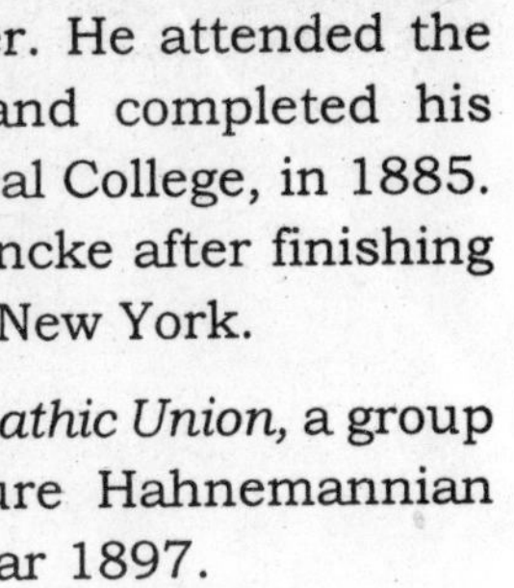

According to Julia M. Green, MD, "Close did not know himself. He seemed to wear a gentle armor of protection, and look out on the world from behind it."

Look behind the obstacles you face in life. They may prove to be windows of opportunity.

SECTION-D .... Page 67 to 94

D-1 ***Dr. Daftari, K.L.***
(Born: 22-11-1880 / Died: 19-02-1956) 68

D-2 ***Dr. Das, Rai Bahadur Bishambar***
(Born: 21-03-1891 / Died: 12-07-1965) 69

D-3 ***Dr. De, D.N.*** (Born: 1877 / Died: 19-09-1943).........70

D-4 ***Dr. Dev, Khan Chand*** (Died: 1941)..........................71

D-5 ***Dr. Desai, Maganlal B.***
(Born: 1906 / Died: 1977) 72

D-6 ***Dr. Dewey, Willis A.***
(Born: 25-10-1858 / Died: 01-04-1938) 74

D-7 ***Dr. Dhawale, Laxman Dinchura***
(Born: 21-07-1884 / Died: 10-12-1960) 75

D-8 ***Dr. Dudgeon, Robert Ellis***
(Born: 17-03-1829 / Died: 18-09-1904) 76

D-9 ***Dr. Dunham, Carroll***
(Born: 29-10-1828 / Died: 18-02-1877) 83

D-10 ***Dr. Dutt, Rajendra Lall***
(Born: 1818 / Died: 05-06-1889) 94

Dr. K.L. Daftari

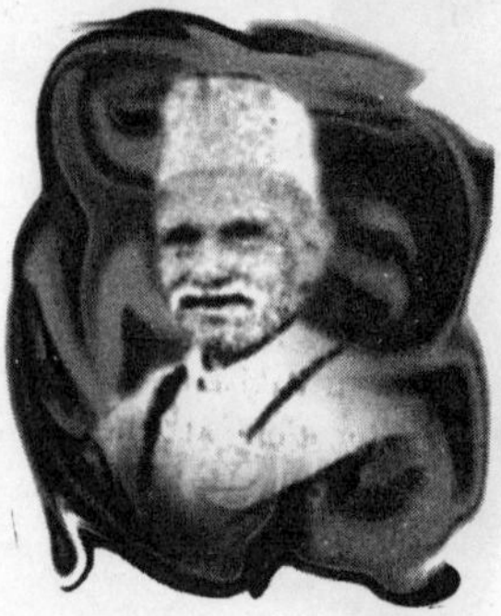

Born : 22-11-1880 Died : 19-02-1956

Dr. Keshav Laxman Daftari was born on November 22, 1880. He learnt Sanskrit, Mathematics and Astronomy from Shri S. K. Barlingay. He graduated in Arts and Law and joined the Bar in the year 1905. He discarded legal practice and joined the national non-cooperation movement. He pursued his *Researches* in 'Hindu Astronomy' and 'Ancient History' which won for him wide acclaim and for this brilliant work, he was awarded the honorary degree of D. Litt. by Nagpur University. He also studied Ayurveda. He was deeply impressed by the logic of Hahnemann and took to the practice of Homoeopathy as a profession. He was a member of the Galendar Committee appointed by the Government of India. Dr. K. D. Daftari was a pioneer in the field of Homoeopathy in Vidarbha region of India. In 1950 he became the first Chairman of the Board of Homoeopathic and Biochemic Systems of Medicine in the erstwhile Madhya Pradesh State. He has written several books on Homoeopathy. He died on Feb. 19, 1956.

Dr. Rai Bahadur Bishambar Das

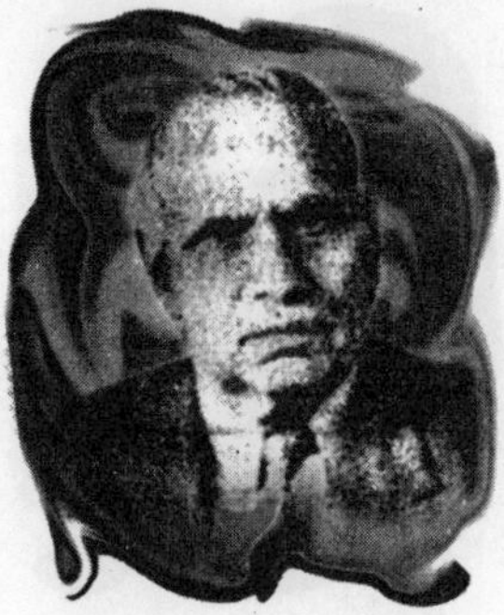

Born : 21-03-1891 **Died : 12-07-1965**

Rai Bahadur Bishambar Das was born on March 21, 1891 in a small village of Ludhiana District of Punjab.

Starting from a modest situation in the Central Secretariat of the Government of India he rose to a high position and became so popular that, to recognise his services to the ailing patients a road has been named after him, in New Delhi.

With no pretention of high academic attainment, ai Bahadur Bishambar Das was primarily a self-made and self-made and self-taught man. His command over English was a high order. He will be long remembered for his wit, and sense or humanity. His zeal for philanthropic led him to learn Homoeopathic from his *gurus* in his spare time. He started independent practice in Homoeopathy in early twenties. His devotion coupled with the passion of public service made Homoeopathy his second profession. He was one the pioneers, who made homoeopathic treatment popular in the country. Working with a missionary zeal, he gave free treatment and medicines to the ailing hundreds who thronged his Charitable Dispensary. He also imparted training to upcoming homoeopaths. Hopless cases found success in his healing touch. His reputation survives and hundreds of patients daily visit the Dişpensary established by him.

In order to make homoeopathic way of treatment popular and within reach of even the poorest of the poor, he wrote the book 'Select Your Remedy', which has a basis of his 45 years experience.

He died in New Delhi on July 12, 1965 at the age of 74.

Section-D : Dr. Das, R.B.B.

Dr. D.N. De

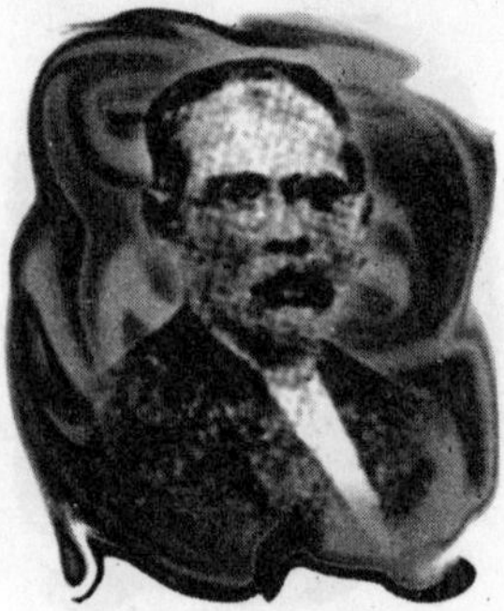

Born : 1877 **Died : 19-09-1943**

Dr. D.N. De, L.M.S., was one of the highly respected homoeopaths and teachers. He founded the Dunham College of Homoeopathy in 1927 and handed over the same to a registered public body in 1937. He expired on September 19, 1943 at the age of 60. His college was later renamed as the D.N. De Homoeopathic Medical College and Hospital to honour his memory.

Section-D : Dr. De, D.N.

Dr. Khan Chand Dev

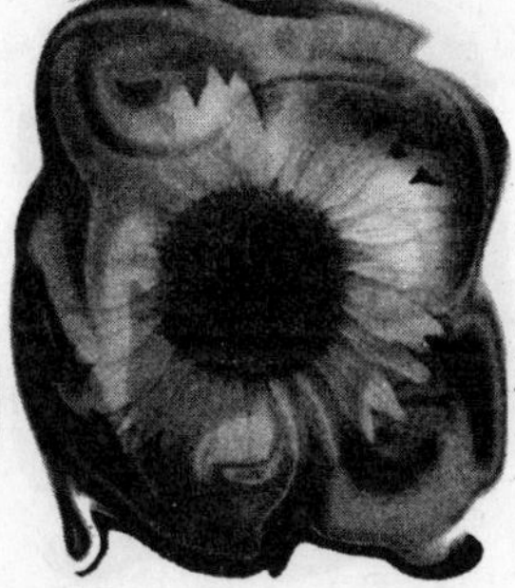

Died : 1941

Late Dr. K. Chand Dev was one of the pioneers of Homoeopathy in the pre-partitioned Punjab and had practiced in Lahore for many years till his death in 1941.

After graduating in medicine from Punjab, Dr. Khan Chand Dev went to U.S.A. and joined the University of Chicago in 1910; after obtaining his M.D. degree he worked as a House Physician in one of the American hospitals and returned to India towards the end of 1914.

After returning to India, he started his practice in the old city of Lahore.

Dr. Maganlal B. Desai

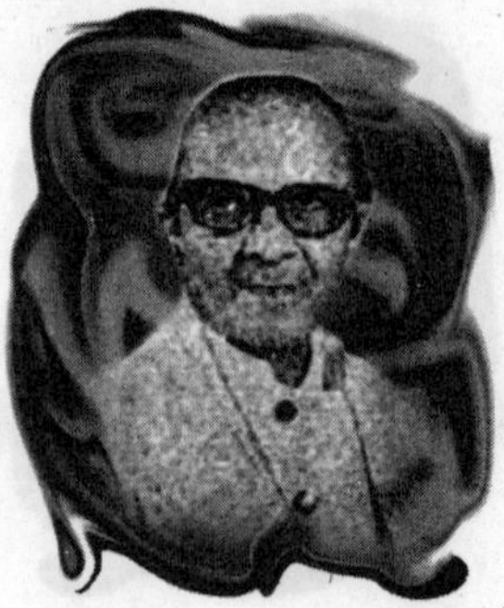

Born : 1906 Died : 1971

Dr. Maganlal Desai was born in 1906 after graduating from the Regular Homoeopathic College in Calcutta in 1928. He practised Homoeopathy for 42 years most actively till his end in 1971. After practising in Calcutta for 12 years, he shifted his activity to Surat, Bombay and Navsari, frequently commuting between these centres. He treated several hundreds of families for many long years taking complete charge of them and putting them exclusively under homoeopathic care whatever their illness. Therefore his observations will carry much weightage.

Even in his early years he found himself more successful by repeating the doses even in high potencies.

In his narration of cases, Dr. Maganlal Desai exudes a confidence which no doubt resulted from his genuine success in therapeutic work. It can be seen that in his method of selection of remedy, emphasis is mainly on the background of the case which he relates to a general concept of power of the remedy homoeopathically visualised and therapeutically confirmed. The theorem is fully proved, when in his cases by striking to the bare threads of conditions and symptoms in the past history in selection of remedy, he succeeds in brining back the manifestation of old symptoms accompanied by cure of most difficult conditions. He writes: "This method of understanding the given condition in the patient will automatically put an end to the crude and mechanical way of repertorising with the total of available symptoms, all and sundry... It will be quite clear that our patient has to pass through a series of conditions or stages while eradicating the disease-condition by

Section-D : Dr. Desai, Maganlal B.

way of elimination. This idea puts end to the miracle one doses shot, which simply effects a palliation or a deviation to something else or a temporary surface management of the ailment. The proper understanding of the disease-condition can enable us to predict the series of situations that may intervene during the cure."

"Again he, in this presentation, points out in his Zinc cases that failure to repeat the medicine may be the cause of failure in securing a cure. This is very important observation. Like Hahnemann, he desires to be judged by results when he states. Even if this reasoning or explanation does not look convincing at this juncture I may mention again that these facts and conclusions are drawn from long experience of cases dealt with successfully in a vast practice and therefore they merit study and acceptance (after proper testing)."

Dr. Willis A. Dewey

Born : 25-10-1858

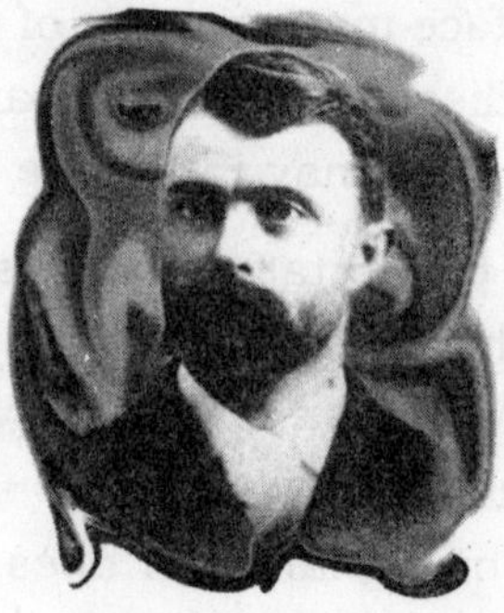

Died : 01-04-1938

Willis A. Dewey, M.D., was born on the 25th of October, 1858. He was a native of Middlebury, Vermout. He graduated from New York Homoeopathic Medical College, in 1880. He did his internship at Ward's Island Homoeopathic Hospital. In 1884 he went to California. He was the professor of anatomy and then in the chair of materia medica at the Homoeopathic Medical College of San Francisco.

He worked as an editor of *The California Homoeopath* from 1888 to 1892. In 1894 he returned back to teach in New York. In 1896 he accepted the chair of medica medica at the University of Michigan at Ann Arbor.

He contributed to homoeopathic literature by writing many books. He wrote *Essentials of Homoeopathic Materia Medica, Essentials of Homoeopathic Therapeutics, and Practical Homoeopathic Therapeutics.* He also worked together with William Boericke on *The Twelve Tissue Salts.*

Section-D : Dr. Dewey, Willis A.

Dr. Laxman Dinchura Dhawale

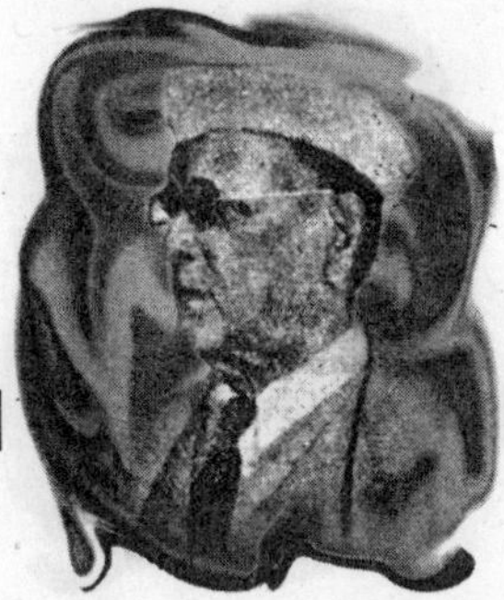

Born : 21-07-1884 **Died : 10-12-1960**

Dr. L.D. Dhanwale was born at bhandara on July 21, 1884. He took his B. A. degree of the allahabad University from the Morris College in 1908. He then became a tutuor in Pathology and later on an Honorary Physician at the K. E. M. Hospital, Bombay. He was a very thoroughgoing and hard task master. Once his father became seriously ill with a Carbuncle on the back. He obtained a copy of allen's 'Handbook of Materia Medica' and managed to find the right remedy. Cure, through slow, soon followed. He then became a convert to Homoeopathy. His homoeopathic leanings brought him into conflict with his superiors. He was a selfmade homoeopathic physican and knew well the difficulties that beset the path of self-made homoeopaths. He, therefore, established the Homoeopathic Post-graduate Association in 1931. He also wrote two booklets: *'The Difficulties in Homoeopathic Practice'* and *'Homoeopathic — Its Principles and Tenets'*.

He was a past-master in the clinical use of the Card Repertory and his Introduction to the 6th editioin of Boger's 'General Analysis' helped to popularise the work. He was appointed by the Government of India in 1948 on the Homoeopathic Enquiry Committee. He was the first Hony. Physician and Superintendent of the Govt. Homoeopathic Hospital, Bombay. He took ill in Feb. 1959 and passed away on Dec. 10, 1960.

He was the founder president of Homoeopathic Post-graduate Association Bombay; Member of Govt. of India Homoeopathic Enquiry Committee, 1948; Hon. Chief Medical Officer and Hon. Physician, Govt. Homeopathic Hospital, Bombay. He conducted the first Homoeopathic Seminar for Ceylon Homoeopathic Society in Colombo.

Dr. Robert Ellis Dudgeon

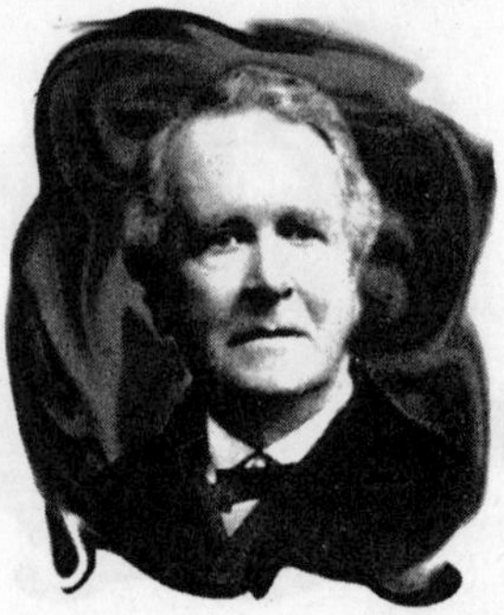

Born : 17-03-1829

Died : 08-09-1904

BIRTH

He was born in a country house in the outskirts of Edingburgh on 17th March, 1829, which is a very auspicious day in Christian theology and is known as Saint Patrick's day.

CHILDHOOD & EDUCATION

He was educated at the Extra Academic Medical School and the University of Edinburgh.

In 1839 he obtained his surgeon's diploma. As per the existing rules he was not allowed to sit for university examination because of his younger age. So he spent two years time chiefly in Paris attending ECOLE de MEDICINE and the hospitals attending to the lectures and clinic of important physicians like Velpeau, Andral, Civiale, Maisonneuve, Louise, Piorry and others.

He returned to Edinburgh and passed his M.D. examination from the Edinburgh University on the 1st of August, 1841.

He went to Vienna and passed a semester and was greatly benefitted by the internationally famous medical men like Skoda, Rokitansky, Hebra, Heller and Jaeger.

In Vienna his fellow students were Drysdale, Russell and Fisher, who all became legendary figures of British homoeopathy, nay, the world homoeopathy. His another fellow student was Wilde, who afterwards became Sir William and did great service to homoeopathy by truthfully stating its successes in cholera in his book on Austria.

They were very close to each other and used to dine together frequently at a favourite restaurant. Drysdale, Fisher and Russel were almost every day studying homoeopathic treatment at Fleischmann's hospital. Dudgeon personally was not interested in homoeopathy at this particular time.

He went to Berlin to study Eye and Ear Diseases under Jungken and Kramer, and Organic Chemistry under Simon. These teachers had a world-wide name and fame for their spcialised knowledge in their respective fields.

Dudgeon spent some time in Dublin to acquire further knowledge and worked under Graves, Stokes (of Cheyne-Stokes fame), Corrigan, Mars and others. They are all famous names in the field of clinical medicine.

MEDICAL PRACTICE & CONVERSION

He settled in medical practice at Liverpool which was the residence of his father. Dr. Drysdale was also practicing in Liverpool and used to insist Dudgeon to take interest in homoeopathy.

In 1843 THE BRITISH JOURNAL OF HOMOEOPATHY was started by Drysdale, Russell and Black although there were hardly a dozen of homoeopathic physician in the United Kingdom at that time. Drysdale used to request Dudgeon to translate articles from German language into English and thus in Dudgeon's own words, "he learnt a good deal about the new system and gradually became a thorough believer."

Vienna in those days was in the hey day of homoeopathic fervour and a vast deal of invaluable work was being done in the way of proving new drugs and reproving old medicines. The homoeopathic societies used to publish valuable articles in their periodicals.

On Drysdale's advice Dudgeon went to Vienna to see homoeopthic practice of Fleischmann in Gumpendorf Hospital and came in contact with Madeen, Hilbers and Macleod. His family and that of Madden used to live together and they spent much time studying homoeopathy jointly and critically. The important homoeopathic physicians of Vienna were Wurmb, Watzke, Gerstel, Zlatarovich, Nehrer and others. He returned to England and started homoeopathic practice in London in 1851 and next year he joined the Editorial Board of the BRITISH JOURNAL OF HOMOEOPATHY, which was in its fourth volume. He joined in place of Black who had withdrawn after the first volume. He remained with the journal till 1884 when the publication ceased for some time.

The journal was haunted by a tragic fate from the beginning.

Russell severed his connections in 1858 and Atkins joined the editorial staff in 1859 whose connections ended in 1861 and in 1863 Richard Hughes joined as an editor and by 1877 Dudgeon and Hughes were left alone after the retirement of Drysdale. Dr. J.H. Clarke joined the journal in 1883 and thus another triumvirate came to work together.

HIS OTHER ACTIVITIES

A few years after the death of Hahnemann *The Central Society of German Homoeopaths* decided to construct a monument of Hanemann at Coethen, for which Rummel was appointed as a treasurer and the Duke of Anhelt-Coethen had promised a liberal contribution. Since Dudgeon considered Coethen a dull little town and Hahnemann's connection with it was purely accidental and transitory, he raised his voice against it. Ultimately Leipzig was decided as the site of monument and for this Dudgeon had to collect the extra funds from British homoeopaths to meet the extra expenses. The occasion was attended by many important physicians and disciples of Hahnemann. Dr. A. Lutze, who practiced in Coethen, constructed a monument also at Coethen at his own expense.

He was instrumental in founding the Hahnemann Hospital and School of Homoeopathy of Bloomsburg Square, with which was connected the Hahnemann Medical Society, where eminent homoeopaths were involved as teachers. Dr. Curie taught Therapeutics, Dr. J. Epps Materia Medica and Dudgeon, himself, Theory and Practice of Homoeopathy.

One of his greatest contribution was his fight against the Draft Medical Bill of 1858, which in response to the agitation of allopaths wanted to regulate the affairs of medical schools and colleges and had made provisions for rejecting the candidates who had any connection with and leaning towards homoeopathy. The famous case is that of Harvey who, in his final stages of examination, was asked to give a written declaration in the name of his honour that he will not practice homoeopathy which he refused and he was not allowed to complete his examination and obtain his degrees. Dudegeon wrote, "The bill if passed in its actual form would allow any examining body to exact similar declarations from candidates and homoeopathy would thus be practically extinguished in this country."

The bill was already passed in the House of Commons and was at the point of being passed in the House of Lords and, if not ammended, would become a Law.

Dudgeon spear-headed the opposition to the bill and with the help of the great benefactors of homoeopathy like Lord Ebury, Mr. William Cowper (later Lord Mount Temple) introduced a Clause no. XXIII which read as follows:

"In case it shall appear to the General Council that an attempt has been made by any body entitled under the act to grant Qualifications, to impose upon any candidate offering himself for examination an obligation to adopt or refrain from adopting the practice of any particular Theory of Medicine or Surgery as a test or condition of admitting him to Examination or granting a Certificate, it shall be lawful for the said Council to represent the same to Her Majesty's most Honourable Privy Council, and the said Privy Council may there upon issue an Injunction to such body so acting directing them to desist from such Practice, and in the event of their not complying therewith then to order that such body shall cease to have the power of conferring any Right to be registered under this act so long as they shall continue such Practice."

And thus a great catastrophe approaching the young healing art was averted.

Another dedicated fight was given by Dudgeon in case of the infirmary of consumption in London, whose majority of the allopathic staff wanted to remove Dr. Jagielski and Dr. Marsh for using homoeopathic medicine in the infirmary. The approached Dudgeon for help. This institution was ruled by a powerful managing committee where members were called Governors and one of the qualifications to be a member (or Governor) was to donate a very large amount of money to the fund of the institution. Dudgeon donated a very large amount of money from his own purse and became one of the Governors of the institution. The battle of wits started and Dudgeon entered into a prolonged battle against conspiracies, cunningness, selfishness and oppression, and won the battle. Seven of the members of staff resigned and soon new staff from homoeopaths and liberal minded allopaths were recruited. The

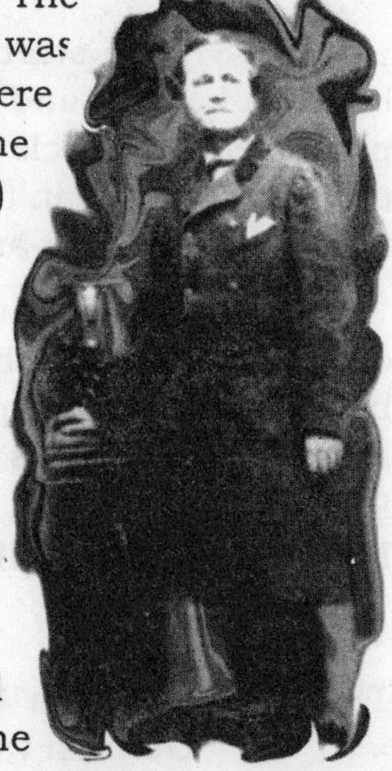

TIMES newspaper of London carried a column ODIUM MEDICUM for six weeks and important physicians from both systems of medicine took part in the controversies. The whole matter was edited by J.H. Clarke and was published by British Homoeopathic Society.

Dudgeon's one more contribution was the founding of Homoeopathic League in 1887 which included homoeopathic physicians and the lay-men sympathiser of homoeopathy to educate the public about the new system and to remove the misconception that Hahnemann's method was only a quackery. The League published 36 popular tracts forming 3 volume which proved very useful in spreading correct knowledge of homoeopathy among the people. This move became so popular and effective that allied associations were formed in France and Spain and many of the tracts were translated into Spanish, French and Italian, and were reproduced in American periodicals and were extensively circulated in India and Australia.

He made an innovation in the use of microscope for examining a considerable quantity of any fluid at a time and his works were published and appreciated in the Quarterly Journal of Microscopic Science.

He was the discoverer of the DIVING GLASSES with which the vision in seabathing or under sea diving is improved. His findings were read before International Ophthalmic Congress of 1872 and was included in the transactions of that Congress. His explanation of the mechanism of Accommodation led to an animated debate in the end of which he was proved to be correct.

In 1873 he started a crusade against the unclean swimming-baths in London and inspected each one of them except 2 or 3, and published an article in The British Journal of Homoeopathy and then published it in the form of a pamphlet. This demonstration led to a reorganisation and better sanitation of these swimming baths.

His most famous discovery of innovation was the preparation of a pocket sized sphygmograph which was mildly opposed in the beginning by the allopaths but later on described and photographed in most of the books on physiology and pathology.

LITERARY CONTRIBUTION

Translations

1849 : Dudgeon translated lots of homeopathic writings from German to English and wrote many himself. Many of his articles are not easily available. Hence, this list of his literary contributions is incomplete.

Hahnemann's Organon of Medicine, 5th German edition, pp. 339. In the end of the book he added an Appendix which "gives a detailed history of the origin, growth and propers of each aphorism and adds some needful explanatory notes".

1851 : Hahnemann's Lesser writings, pp. 784. He collected 51 writings of Hahnemann of pre-homoeopathic and homoepathic period and translated them.

1880 : Materia Medica Pura, complete in 2 Vols, Vol. I p. 718, 37 medicines; Vol. II, p. 709, 30 medicines.

Original Writings

1851 : His Translator's Preface of Hahnemann's writings. This is a wonderful summary of 20 writings both original and translations, essays and books, of Hahnemann which are not included in the Lesser writings.

1852 : Biographical Sketch of Hahnemann, p. 53.

1854 : Lectures on Theory and Practice of Homoeopathy, p. 565.

1870 : The Human Eye : Its Optical Considerations.

1891 : Address to the International Homoeopathic Congress, 1891. He has been acclaimed as the best of the English translators of the works of Hahnemann and he himself wrote, "My contributions to homoeopathic literature are too numerous to mention, but perhaps my chief claim of remembrance by the homoeopathic world is as the translator of all Hahnemann's homoeopathic works except CHRONIC DESEASES and many of his pre-homoeopathic works."

HIS LITERARY STYLES

Dr. W. Von Baun describes Dudgeon's literary styles as "interesting, racy, humorous but modest style."

PROFESSIONAL ACHIEVEMENTS

1. He was twice chosen as the President of the British Homoeopathic Society and once British Homoeopathic Congress.

2. He was chosen as the President of the International Homoeopathic Congress at Atlantic City.

   Dudgeon writes about himself "I have been engaged in almost every controversy on homoeopathy in the medical and lay periodical."

"I believe I am the first and only avowed partisan of homoeopathy who has defended the method of Hahnemann in the London Medical Society."

CHARACTER

Even in his seventies he was "hale and hearty" and did his professional work without fatigue, played golf whole day, once a week, went for gouse shooting every year, in the month of August for 3 weeks and used to take long swing every day. He was very fond of shooting patridges and pheasants.

DEMISE

In the morning session of The British Homoeopathic Congress on July, 1, Dudgeon told his friends that he was troubled with a skin irritation which interfered with sleep and gave him a feeling of general illness. He never left his house after this date. This trouble developed into a abnormal form of pemphigus which undermined his vital power and inspite of his mental faculties remaining unimpaired, he sank from weakness.

At the age of 85 years on 8th of September, 1904, he passed away peacefully without pain, without any complain and without any disturbance.

SOURCE MATERIALS

R.E. Dudgeon : My Autobiography published in the monthly Homoeopathic Review, October, 1904, p. 577.

: The Hahnemannian Monthly, 1892.

: Homoeo Rays, February to May, 1976.

Dr. Carroll Dunham

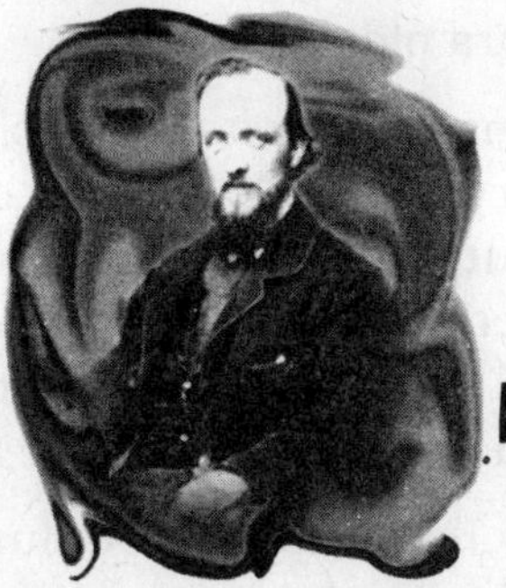

Born : 29-10-1828

Died : 18-02-1877

"His life was gentle; and the elements so mixed in him, that Nature might stand up and say to all the world — This Was A Man."

The memory of this great and good man is enshrined in the work he accomplished on earth, as well as in the hearts of all who came within the circle of his wise and helpful benevolence.

"Si monumentum quaries, or circumspice!" Although no words can enrich such a record, they may serve even in a fragmentary review, to present the leading traits of this noble life with sufficient distinctness for profitable study.

ANCESTORS & FAMILY

The families of his father Edward Wood Dunham and mother Maria Smyth Parker were prominent old residents of New Brunswick in the state of New Jersey. Mr. Dunham was a successful merchant and was known for his intelligence, energy, methodical habits and success in business. In 1820 he shifted his family from New Brunswick to New York and retired in 1853, a rich, contented and successful man and became the President of Corn Exchange Bank.

Mrs. Maria Symth was distinguished by her gentleness, prudence and firmness.

BIRTH

Carroll Dunham was born on October 29, 1828 in New York. He was the youngest of the four sons of Mr. Edward Wood and Mrs. Maria Smyth Dunham.

CHILDHOOD & EDUCATION

Carroll's mother died during the cholera epidemic of 1832, when he was only 4 years old.

As a child he was marked as a docile, cheerful and bright boy who was very particular about the feelings of others. Although he was a healthy child but he avoided the rough sports and was described by his elder brother as "Always looking into things with an eager desire to know all about their qualities and uses." He was more fond of books than play.

He graduated with honours from Columbia College in 1847 and then commenced the study of medicine.

In 1850 he received his M.D. from the College of Physicians and Surgeons then located in Crosby Street of New York.

He was well known for his patience, happy temperament and willingness to help and a select band of followers used to gather everyday around him to hear the explanation of the subjects taught in the class that day.

CONVERSION TO HOMOEOPATHY

He was cured of a serious and dangerous malady in which the best allopathic treatment failed and was subsequently cured by a homoeopath. This impressed him and his father. He started reading homoeopathic literatures and comparing homoeopathic result with that of allopathy. His findings impressed him further. After completing his studies he went to Philadelphia to see Dr. Constantine Hering, who was then the high-priest of homoeopathy in U.S.A. He learned much about homoeopathy and more over, in his own words, "gained the most helpful, generous and genial friend ever made."

His father's wish was to let him see the medical world of Europe and acquire as much knowledge of new techniques & methods in medicine as far possible and Dr. Carroll Dunham was despatched on a long tour of Europe.

In Dublin he served as an internee in the Lying-in-hospital and was allowed to investigate the stokes treatment of fevers in Meath Hospital. In Dublin he received a dissecting wound which nearly ended his career, but a homoeopathic physician cured him again when the Resident Surgeon had given up all hopes of any help.

He went to Paris and came in contact with many eminent allopathic physicians like Bouillard, Velpeau, Trousseaue and he regularly visited the homoeopathic hospital under the guidance of Dr. Tessier. From Paris he went to Berlin and then to Vienna where he remained several months attending to the hospital clinics of Wurmb and the lectures of Kaspar on Materia Medica. Then he went to Munter to visit Boenninghausen who received him cordially and in turn was impressed by Dr. Dunham's industry and intelligence. He prophesied a bright future for young Carroll. Dr. Dunham remained there long enough to see numerous cases being cured by the distinguished old guard and could observe his method of examining the patient and prescribing for them. He literally and liberally availed himself with the foreign culture and education. Dr. Dunhan turned his steps towards his homeland.

MARRIAGE

In 1854, Dr. Dunham married Miss Harriet E. Kellogg, daughter of Edward and Esther F. Kellogg, a woman of rare beauty and intelligence. She was a helping companion and her co-operation in his arduous labours helped him immensely in his work. They were so close and deep in love that they used to tell their children — as if to prepare them for the future — that should one parent die, they must expect the other soon to follow, a prediction which was literally fulfilled, as in less than a year after Dr. Dunham's death, his wife was laid by his side in Greenwood.

MEDICAL PRACTICE

After returning back to America, Dr. Dunham started his practice in Brooklyn. Very soon he acquired fame for his behaviour, and care of the patient. His ability and success were so marked that Dr. P.P. Wells, an esteemed friend and family physician of the Dunham's family said, "He was always like my friend and never my pupil".

Due to severe illness he had to change his residence to Newburgh, New York from Brooklyn in 1858. This time he was in need of rest and decided not to resume practice until fully restored. But the remarkable success which attended his prescriptions were pressed upon him with an urgency not to be denied, brought many other to him and thus, inspite of the delicate state of his health, he soon became very busy in practice.

After six years' stay in Newburgh he again got an attack of

cardiac rheumatism and was removed to New York for a short time, where leading specialists of old school could not show any light of hope regarding his survival. Then Dr. Dunham himself sought advice of Dr. Hering who prescribed a single remedy which completely cured Dr. Dunham from his illness. Thus his own case, more than once, illustrated the soundness of this unique and noble system of medicine, which he often advocated, "a single remedy and if possible, a single dose." Within a short period he changed his residence and settled in Irvington on the banks of river Hudson, which became his home untill his death. However, he continued an office and consulting practice in New York to which he used to attend on certain days of the week.

HIS CHARACTER

Dr. Dunham was very fond of his father and there existed a rare degree of affection and confidence between the two. During his long absence from home he used to write daily letters to his father and this probably helped him to acquire the habit of clear and terse expression which is a characteristic of his writings. Even his longest articles were rarely re-written.

He was very jolly and cheerful. Wherever this young physician went he was sure to make warm and constant friends many of whom were eminent in the homoeopathic world and he kept up a life-long correspondence with them.

He was very affectionate, truthful and energetic. His demeanour towards his fellows was marked by that same modest reserve — far removed from timidity — which was a prominent characteristic throughout his whole life.

He was intelligent, bright and a very capable student. By his greater natural ability he outstripped his fellow friends during his student life, to whom he used to explain daily class lectures.

In all the relations of life, he proved himself as a noble gentlemen. He was a true and tender husband, and a kind and faithful father.

It is not easy to judge and analyze the character of a genius like Dr. Carroll Dunham, but we can always say that his character was like a clear crystal, many-sided and transparent throughout his whole harmonious life. His consecration of himself to a noble ideal of duty was so evident that a friend of his, either of a few weeks or of life-time, would form essentially, the same judgement of him, differing only in the degree in which they would comprehend the nobility of his nature.

DEMISE

In 1858 he was compelled, by a severe illness, to shift to Newburgh New York for complete seclusion and rest. He had to discontinue his practice. But his success in one or two urgent cases brought a large number of sick men to his door. The sought rest was denied and the discontinued practice grew itself against his wishes and health. After six years in Newburgh he suffered an attack of cardiac rheumatism again and was removed for a short time, to New York. The prognosis according to the leading cardiologists was that he could not servive long. He sought the advice of Dr. Constrantine Hering who after a careful study of his symptoms prescribed a dose of *Lithium carbonicum,* which promptly cured him. He again shifted his residence to Irvington, on the banks of the river, Hudson, and made his permanent home there but kept an office of consulting practice in New York, which he used attend on certain days of the week.

His health compelled him several times to change the scene and climate. He visited Europe thrice in the pursuit of health, and also Nassau and other foreign health resorts.

His feeble health and overstrain, especially by the odd hours of working for the world convention marked irreparable damage to his body. He was bedstricken on December 2nd, 1876.

A mild irritating cough, irregular fever, relapse of rheumatism in slight degrees all were aggravated after his strenuous involvement in convention of 1876.

He breathed his last, in his 49th year, on February 18th, 1877. Dr. Joslin wrote, "though his death was obviously caused by exhausted vitality, consequent on his labours in connection with the World's Homoeopathic Convention, and though the nervous system must be looked upon as the main seat of trouble, still the mind remained clear to the last and was never clouded during any period of illness. " Dr. P.P. Wells also said that "he died of no disease, but from exhaustion produced by excessive and protracted labour."

CONTRIBUTIONS

During his last visit to Europe even with his indifferent health he sought the corporation of the foreign physicians in his project of a "WORLD HOMOEOPATHIC CONVENTION" in June, 1876 at Philadelphia.

He was elected the President of the world convention for 1876. It has been claimed that he performed his duties as a President with courtesy and fine fact that few who were present will ever forget. About it he himself wrote to one of his friends, "of course, I have convention on the brain. I eat, sleep and live it and have put source of my best blood into it. But hope to have some life, when all is over."

After the demise of Dr. Duntam, his wife spent her of time and energy in collecting and publishing his numerous but scattered articles into a book form.

Mrs. Dunham gave a vivid detail of the last days of Dr. Dunham. She writes, "A mind so acute as Dr. Dunham's could not have death approach his body and he was unaware of it. Neither could a mind so exalted fail to submit tranquality to an inevitable fate, from which the spirituality of his life took away all fear. He passed from one room in his father's house to another. He said, "I do not see my way through this illness and at the end of the seventh week, a month before he died, he with perfect tranquility slip into my grave. I shall go on in this way two weeks longer, and then I shall slip into my grave. And again I shall go on in this way through the minute week, and then I shall go to Greenwood." About five days before the last morning, I noticed a change in his complexion, this deepened and became more permanent every day until the last moment. Up to that time he had wished the room cool and after few hours he frequently asked if it was warm enough. Sunday morning about eight o'clock, he asked the temperature. He said "There is an unfriendly feeling in the air you better light the fire." He lay and looked into the flame, saying 'That is very pleasant', and he watched us feed the flame, and seemed to enjoy the cheery influence, speaking now and then. And so he passed away a little before nine o'clock, without any struggle. He peacefully ceased to breathe."

Dr. Dunham was a voluminous writer, though he never concentrated his energies on the production of a single large work. He began to contribute articles to the medical journals when in Europe in 1852, and continued to do steadily for twentyfive years, until death ended his labors. He devoted his efforts principally to the elaboration and perfection of the materia medica; though many of his writings are of a miscellaneous character, being reports,

---

Section-D : Dr. Dunham, Carroll

reviews, clinical cases, public addresses, lectures, monographs and translations, the most notable of the last being Boenninghausen's work on whooping cough. But these productions of his pen are not to be classed among the higher or more ephemeral growth of medical literature. His faculty of giving his best powers to whatever he found to do, great or small, confers a permanent value on all that he wrote. He touched no subject without revealing something new and instructive, while the confidence he inspires in his statements, the judicial impartiality with which he treats matters in debate, and the lucid and namely language which he employs, give a rare zest to his compositions. There was no flaw in the fabric of his thoughts. He never said an unkind word or a silly one, and his opponents (he had no enemies) always admitted that his criticisms were just and manly. Every utterance of his was as perfect as the workings of that noble mind could make it. All his speeches, all his writings, all his labors were, in every part, symmetrical; for all were born of his earnest desire to "do good and communicate." Many of these contributions to our literature appeared in the "American Homoeopathic Review", of which he was editor for some years; but all the prominent journals of our school, with scarcely an exception, were frequently enriched by articles from his pen. Besides his published writings, he maintained a more or less active correspondence with professional friends at home and abroad; in this way his great influence was more widely and thoroughly felt, in the advancement of medical Science and specially of homoeopathic therapeutics.

Always subordinating his private interests to his elevated sense of duty. Dr. Dunham never sought titular honors or any public recognition of what he was or what he had done. But honors found him out and he was, at various times, elected to high positions in many learned and scientific societies, both foreign and domestic testimonials to his reputation as a physician and a scholar which were fully deserved.

When the death of Dr. Dunham was announced, general and profound was the sense of an irreparable loss, that the whole homoeopathic profession rose up as one man, both in this country and in Europe, to give utterance to their sorrow to do honor to his memory and to commemorate his character and services. Every one felt that we had lost "our best man". Special memorial meetings were called in many of our cities; all our societies paid their mournful tribute to his worth; obituary notices from the pens of our most distinguished men appeared in all our journals. Not even the death of Hahnemann stirred up such depths of grief for Dunham, stricken down in the prime of his manhood, was nearly as widely known and admired and was vastly most beloved. Perhaps we cannot give a better ideas of the man, and of the impression which he made, than by quoting from some of the remarks and addresses which were then made as an offering to his memory.

A life long friend remarked, "He was many-sided to such an extent as I have never seen in any other man. His learning was surprising, his literary culture great, and his modesty great as either. He spoke the languages of modern Europe as his own. His insight into the elements of disease, and into the nature of the agents by which they are cured, was wonderful. He has left an example which may God help us to follow.

Another friend said of him; "Not long after the beginning of our acquaintance, we were associated in the investigation of some professional controversies. I confess I was hardly prepared for the display of clear, discriminating sagacity with which he took up the subject in dispute, and the earnestness with which he pursued the delicate and unpleasant task to a logical conclusion. Most of the member of this society know something of the important part he took in the recognization of our medical college. But few are aware of the amount of arcous labor which he gave to that business or of the peculiar difficulties he surmounted in its accomplishment. His opinions always commanded respect, and usually controlled the course of action. And it may be said, without hesitation, that the existing laws of the state for regulating medical practice and for suppressing quackery owe much of their fair and liberal character to the influence he exerted..... Though the functions of arbitrator or inquisitor were not congenial to his modest and retiring disposition, yet he never hesitated to occupy any position or perform any duty legitimately imposed upon him.... In the social circle, amongst neighbors and friends, his genial nature shone conspicuous. With a vast fund of curious and interesting information, gathered from books and travel, he possessed a rare wit, and a fine appreciation of humor, which gave to his conversation a delightful charm and freshness".

The committee of the New York County Homoeopathic Medical Society, after bearing grateful testimony to his invaluable contributions to the materia medica, in the knowledge and practical application of which he was almost without a peer, speak thus of his qualities: "Possessing intellectual capacities of the highest order, he never exert them for selfish ends, but always for the public good. Pure in his private life, exceptionally modest and retiring in his demeanor, ever gentle and kind, he knew not how to stop to meanness and detraction; generous and large hearted, he was always ready to aid others, and all who were brought in contact with his noble and tender nature were compelled not only to admire and venerate the accomplished physician, but to trust and love the true-hearted Christian man".

From a Western physician we have this testimony "At the meetings of our institute, he was the one who moved about the most quietly, who came and went with the least par de, and who, while he spoke very seldom in debate, always spoke to the purpose. He was the member whose committee never failed to report, and whose papers were always well digested, clear, concise, practical, and ready for the printer. He was the source of appeal for men on both sides of mooted questions. His influence was almost unhounded. He had the skill and tact of a great diplomatist, but these were never used for his own personal purposes. His pen was his sword — the sword of Melancthon and not of Luther, bright, keen, trenchant — but it can truly be said that it "never carried a heart-stain away on its blade".

Another friend said "His life was one of truth and goodness. His name can never be mentioned without awakening feelings of love and reverence. His action in all matters, great or small, was prompted by purity of heart and love of right. By years of devotion to his profession, by his searching investigations, by his lucid writings, by his spotless integrity, and by his sincerity of purpose, he acquired unequaled influence among his colleagues; and I truly believe that Carroll Dunham has done more for the interests of homoeopathy, not only in this city or country, but in the world at large, than any other man since the time of Hahnemann."

His life-long friend Dr. P.P. Wells, said, after his death, "I would willingly have died for him".

One who had known him from his boyhood thus spoke of him "When I pass in review the thirty-five years of our friendship, I can honestly and heartily say, that I do not remember a single world or act of his for which any of his friends need to blush, or which he, now gone to his last account, would wish to be unsaid or undone. The only impatience I ever felt toward him during his long period, arose a few times because his calm, deliberative nature refused to plunge into the arena of medical polemics. But he was so magnanimous, or to use the more expressive saxon word, so large minded, that he could not be partisan; he could not but view both sides of every question at issue, and, as a consequence, he was liberal and generous even to his opponents, always ready to make allowance for the opinions and acts of those who differed with him. He was truly one of the 'blessed peace-makers.' The character of his mind was essentially judicial; approaching a subject impartially he calmly weighed it in all its bearings; and had he been educated for the bar, his keen intellect and sound judgment would have graced the highest hence in the land. Actualed by an earnest love of truth and justice, he was thoroughly unselfish and always subordinated his private interests to the good of the cause with which he was identified. More than this his whole life was devoted, in a most self-sacrificing spirit to the duties which the profession laid upon his willing shoulders; duties and responsibilities which he never refused and which came to him unsought, simply because all recognized his eminent fitness for their discharge. Thus he was often overburdened, and on several occasions his failing health compelled him to break off from all labor, and go abroad to rest and recuperate. But the moment he returned, those labors were resumed; and when, at last exhausted nature succumbed, his death was merely the crowning act of a whole life of self-sacrifice. Though not physically strong, he was a steady worker and close student; and though independent of his income as a practitioner, and possessed of a competence by inheritance, which would, especially in view of his impaired health, have justified him in leading a life of elegant leisure, he accomplished an immense amount of literary labor; more, in fact, than most men, in full health and impelled by necessity could have performed."

"His judgement was so sound, his convictions so sincere, his aims so unselfish, his life so pure, his sympathies so tender he was so free from conceit or arrogance, so modest and obtrusive, so devoid of petty ambitions, so intent on doing his whole duty, so liberal and tolerant towards those who differed with him, that he commanded the respect and worn the affection of all who knew him. He wielded an immense power for good not only by what he actually did, but by the mere force of his example, of a quiet, honest thoughtful life."

"I have spoken of him as unselfish; I may from my private

knowledge, that he was very generous and open-handed to all in need, imparting freely not only of his stores of knowledge, but of his purse. I could recount many acts of kindly charity and timely aid to poor struggling brethren; but I refrain, for he was one of those who never let their right hand known what their left hand gives."

"His unvarying cheerfulness was another marked characteristic, notwithstanding his physical infirmities and his engrossing labour, he always seemed to dwell in a bright and serene stmosphere, full of hope and peace. His very presence was refreshing and inspiring; he went in and out among us, impressing all with the conviction that he was a true man, who had consecrated his life to a novel ideal of duty."

"Yes friends and colleagues, we have lost our noblest and best man, one who was the heart and soul of the highest work done in our profession. In him we lose more than we now know; for 'take him all in all, we never shall look upon his life again.' But those who were so blessed as to call him friend, will always be thankful for his life and example; for such a man as he ennobles not only the age in which he lived, but humanity itself."

Much more might be quoted of the same purport; but these extracts will suffice to show how great and good a man was Carroll Dunham; as true a hero as ever fell in the front of battle, fighting for the right.

We cannot close this brief memorial more fitly than by quoting his parting words to his class, for they strike the key-note of his own life:

"May you have the pleasant consciousness, not only that you have made some permanent additions to the common stock of knowledge for the common good, but also that many men and women have been the happier for your lives."

Dr. Rajendra Lall Dutt

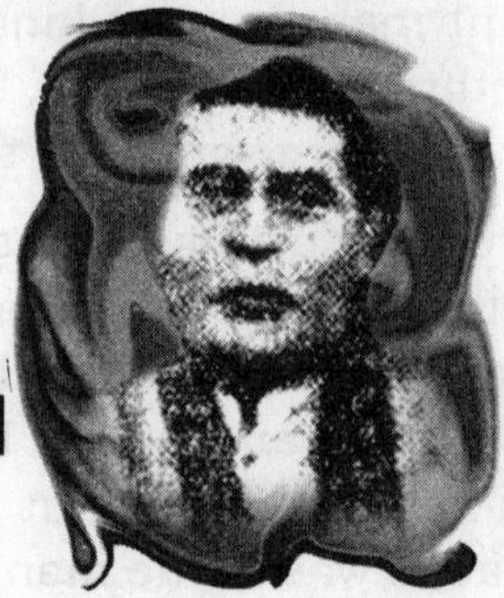

Born : 1818 **Died : 05-06-1889**

If Dr. Mahendra Lal Sircar may be called the fosterer of Indian homoeopathy, Babu Rajendra Lall Dutt may be called the Father of Indian homoeopathy. It was he who converted Dr. Sircar to be a homoeopath. It was Dr. Rajendra Lall Dutt who brought homeopathy into high esteem of the elites of Bengal by curing illustrious luminaries like Pandit Ishwar Chandra Vidyasagar, Raja Sir Radhakanta Dev and score of others.

He was born in the famous Dutt family of Wellingatons Square, Calcutta and amassed immense fortune by dint of his personal talent in honest business and trade and spent the whole of it in various philanthropic works and mostly for homoeopathy. He expired at the age of 71 years on June 5, 1889, leaving homoeopathy on a firm, sound and wide footing.

SECTION-F .... Page 95 to 102

F-1 ***Dr. Farrington, Ernest A.***
(Born: 01-01-1847 / Died: 15-12-1885) 96

F-2 ***Dr. Franz, Karl Gottlab***
(Born: 08-05-1795 / Died: 08-11-1835) 100

Dr. Ernest A. Farrington

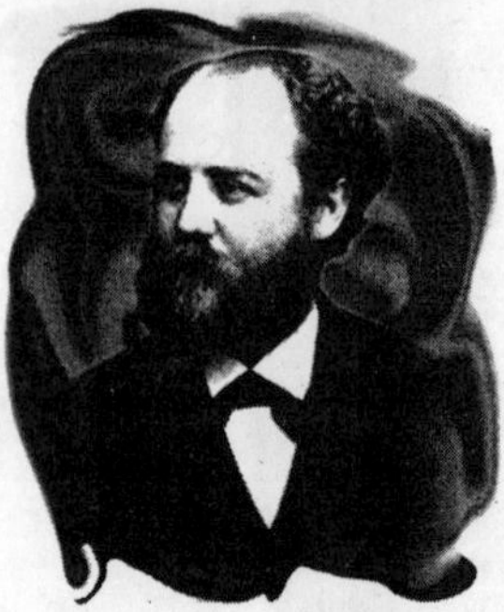

Born : 01-01-1847 **Died : 15-12-1885**

The name of Dr. E.A. Farrington is well known to Homoeopathic world because of his great contribution in the field of Materia Medica. The followers of the homoeopathic system of healing art will be indebted to Farrington for his writings specially for his book on *Clinical Materia Medica.* Farrington's name remains on top of those teachers and authors of materia medica which gave the subject a new dimension, a new vision of application and a new instrument for application.

BIRTH

Ernest A. Farrington was born on 1st of January, 1847 in Brooklyn, a locality then known as Williamburg, in New York.

EDUCATION

His family left Brooklyn for Philadelphia when Farrington was very young and so he received his education there.

Nature had endowed him with sharp perception, exceptional memory, genial manners and a helping nature. He was distinguished as a pupil and popular amongst his school mates. His power to grasp and assimilate facts characterised him as a phenomenal pupil in the eyes of his teachers.

At 19 years of age, he passed from Philadelphia High School breaking all records of previous examinations of the institution. For a long time he was remembered by his teachers for his aptness, clearness of thought and remarkable proficiency.

In the summer of 1866 he visited his birth place in New York city and returned to Philadelphia to resume his studies. In 1866 he matriculated from Homoeopathic Medical School in

---

Section-F : Dr. Farrington, Ernest A.

Pennsylvania, where his intelligence, memory and conscientiousness in addition to religious bent of mind earned him admiration and affection of his fellow students and teachers.

In the March of 1868, he again graduated from Hahnemann Medical College in Philadelphia.

MEDICAL PRACTICE

He started his practice in 1861 at Mount Vernon Street. His studious nature and engagements in practice soon affected his health and so in 1864 he took a short European trip which improved his health.

In the spring of 1869 he was appointed as a lecturer in Forensic Medicine in Hahnemann Medical College. He proved his mettle as versatile, intellectual and competent teacher and within two years he was appointed to the Chair of Pathology & Diagnosis.

In 1874 he was appointed the Professor of Materia Medica, after the resignation of the famous Dr. Guernsey and thus, Farrington attained the dream and aim of his life, because it was Materia Medica which was his cherished field of labor, deepest studies and it was in this subject that his life's work began.

He made deep and analytical studies in the matters of homoeopathic principles, rules, dosage, potency and the content and the teaching methods of materia medica.

Korndoerfer says, "His daily association with Hering quickened his natural desire and he was soon recognised by that master spirit of our school (i.e. Hering) as one well fitted to a place in the highest rank among the expounders of that most intricate science, Materia Medica. Hering was delighted to say — when I am gone, Farrington must finish my materia medica." In fact, Farrington and A. Korndoerfer had assisted Dr. Hering in compiling Condensed Materia Medica (published in 1877) and Farrington revised, enlarged and improved the 3rd edition of the book (published in 1884) after Hering's death in 1881, but his name does not appear among the editors (Drs. C. G. Raue, C. B. Knerr and C. Mohr) but in the Preface with a remark that "we desire to thank Dr. E.A. Farrington for useful suggestions."

MARRIAGE & FAMILY

On 13th of September, 1871 Farrington married Miss Elizabeth Aitkin, who proved to be a woman perfectly suited to his professional and religious inclinations. The couple had three sons and one daughter.

HIS CONTRIBUTIONS & ATTACHMENTS

Not only the admirable quality of Dr. Farrington as a professor promoted homoeopathy he worked as an active worker in various societies for the cultivation of medical science, and his valuable writings and papers in different journals have made homoeopathy rich. His contributions to our literature are of great practical merit and combine completeness of statement, cogency of reasoning and consciousness of expression in a remarkable degree. In latter part of his life he was a contributing editor of the HAHNEMANNIAN MONTHLY for several years.

In 1879 when Hahnemannian Monthly was purchased by the Hahnemannian Club of Philadelphia, he was selected as the sole editor of the journal, but due to impairment of his health and multiplicity of duties he accepted the position of contributing editor.

His writings in materia medica alone consisted about two hundred pages in the Hahnemannian Monthly. The American Journal of Homoeopathic Materia Medica, The North American Journal of Homoeopathy and several other journals received valuable articles from his pen.

For many years he was a member of the committee on drug proving and closely identified with the important Bureau of Materia Medica in Hahnemann Medical College.

Later in 1884, he was appointed as a member of the editorial committee on the new "Cyclopedia of Drug Pathogensy" by the institute.

In the same year, he was selected as a member of the State Society and the American Institute of Homoeopathy.

He was a ready and logical speaker and always heard with marked attention in debates.

His devotion to materia medica was unprecedented. To the study and elucidation of this science he devoted much attention and many complicated problems regarding drug action engaged the best efforts of his mind.

LITERARY CONTRIBUTIONS

1874 : A supplement to Gross, Comparative Materia Medica.

1887 : A Clinical Materia Medica.

1890 : The same; 2nd Edition (some more drug indications are added to this edition).

HIS OTHER LITERARY CONTRIBUTIONS

- Syllabus to Materia Medica.
- Lesser Writings with Therapeutic Hints.
- Editing of Hering's Condensed Materia Medica.
- Co-editing of the Hahnemannian Monthly.

Besides this list, Farrington wrote a large number of valuable and important articles in different prominent journals and periodicals of his time.

DEATH

Farrington was a man of strong and vigorous constitution, which gave him the strength of carrying various labors without serious effects to his health. An attack of minor cold resulted in laryngitis which compelled him to suspend his lectures. Shortly after this he again resumed his college duties and developed severe bronchitis. By the month of April he got some relief. Then he decided to go for a tour in the hope that change may cure him completely. However, he returned after few months with aggravated symptoms. Subsequently his disease progressed and ultimately on 15th of December, 1885 he breathed his last in Philadelphia at the age of 38 years, 11 months and 16 days.

In his death the faculty and students of the Hahnemann Medical College, and Philadelphia Country Homoeopathic Medical Society lost a guide and a source of strength.

SOURCE MATERIALS

1. American Institute of Homoeopathy
2. C. Bartlett : Preface to the first edition: Farrington's Clinical Materia Medica.
3. T.L. Bradford : Bibliography.
4. Aug. Korndoerfer : Professor E.A. Farrington, in the Hahnemannian Monthly, January , 1886.

Dr. Karl Gottlab Franz

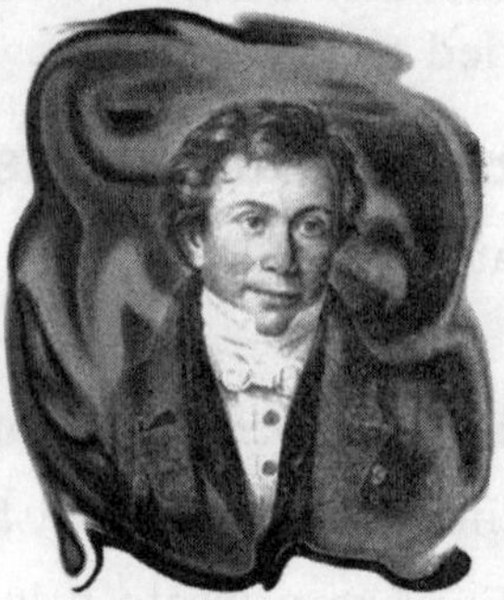

Born : 08-05-1795 **Died : 08-11-1835**

Karl Gottlab Franz was one of the most earnest and ardent followers of Hahnemann. He was one of the earliest who suffered immensely, and was mocked and humiliated by the contemporary medical men. Like many stalwarts of homoeopathy, Dr. Franz was also a convert from allopathic school and he too, like many others has come to the folds of homoeopathy after the cure of his serious ailments.

BIRTH & EARLY EDUCATION

Franz was born in a well-to-do family on 8th of May, 1795 in Plauen in the Royal Saxon Voigtland. His father was a respectable man and a baker by profession.

He finished his high school studies from Plauen High School.

To fulfill his parents' wish he went to Leipzig in 1814 for further studies of theology, though his favourite subjects were botany and medicine.

MEDICAL EDUCATION

He started a trend of changing from Theology to Medicine in general and homoeopathy in particular in Leipzig and was followed by Hartmann and Hornburg who were a year junior to him in class.

But Franz has to discontinue his studies because of his ill health. He was suffering from some very painful ailment as a result of badly treated skin eruptions. On one of his friends advise Franz went to Hahnemann for his treatment and was attracted by the truthfulness and open behaviour of Hahnemann and his new method of treatment whose marvellous result he observed in his

---

Section-F : Dr. Franz, Karl Gottlab

own case. Very soon he became a zealous friend and follower of Hahnemann. He received his medical diploma in 1825.

MEDICAL PRACTICE & HARASSMENTS

Franz started treating patients only some days after he came in contact with Hahnemann. "Although he was made happy on one side by the ever brighter light of the newly gained truth, there was no lack on the other hand of hardships which lay in wait for him on this new and thorny path."

In the year 1820 he was involved by some physicians of Leipzig in a very distressing lawsuit lasting several years, though itended probably for him.

In 1821 his homoeopathic medicine chest was confiscated along with that of Harburg's and was buried publicly in St. Paul's churchyard, at the instigation of Dr. Clarus of Leipzig University.

In 1825 he went to Vienna on the invitation of Countess Von Trautmanns for curing her of her ailments. He stayed there for nine months.

Inspite of all his harassment, humiliations and sufferings he continued to practice homoeopathy till his last days.

FAMILY LIFE

Franz married in the year 1827. He had a very happy and peaceful family life though he had no children.

DEATH

His chronic malady of youth again started giving him troubles. He suffered, unspeakably, from the ailments of liver and bladder. His health was slowly degenerating.

He was relieved of all his pains when he succumbed to his maladies on 8th November, 1835 at the early age of 40 years and 6 months.

CONTRIBUTIONS

Karl Gottlab Franz devoted his whole life to the noble cause of homoeopathy. He worked for and with Hahnemann and became his right-hand man. In experiments with drugs and drug-proving, he did the most laborious job of arranging the symptoms of the drugs in accordance with Hahnemann's previously directed schema.

He used to copy symptoms and arrange them alphabetically according to locations. These were to be done nearly daily. His hard working earnest and honest nature very soon earned him a very respectable place in the eyes of Hahnemann.

Hering says about him "the noble self-sacrificing man".

Franz had a very sound knowledge of Botany. He spared no pains in making himself acquainted with the various indigenous plants and gathered information about them. We owe much to him for it was he who gathered most of the plants from which tinctures were prepared and drug-proving was done.

Though he has published nothing in book form but his devotion, most meticulous single-handed and monotonous labors, sacrifices and contribution can be seen in the pages of Hahnemann's Materia Medica Pura and the homoeopathic journal "Archiv Fur Die Homoeopathische Helkust."

SOURCE MATERIALS

1. Richard Hael — Samuel Hahnemann: His Life and Work, 2 Vols.
2. T.L. Bradford : Life and Letters of Hahnemann.
3. T.L. Bradford : The Pioneers of Homoeopathy.
4. Dr. Mahendra Singh — Samuel Hahnemann: A biographical monument and chronology.
5. North Western Journal of Homoeopathy. Vol. IV, P. 186.
6. Medical Counsellor, 1886, P.240.
7. Hahnemannian Monthly : 1885, P. 175.
8. British Journal of Homoeopathy, 1874. P. 456.

SECTION-G .... Page 103 to 127

G-1 ***Dr. Ghatak, Nilmani***
(Born: 1872 / Died: 19-01-1940) 104

G-2 ***Dr. Ghosh, S.C.***
(Born: 1870 / Died: 1953).......................................107

G-3 ***Dr. Gross, Gustav Wilhelm***
(Born: 06-09-1794 / Died: 18-09-1847)................118

G-4 ***Dr. Guernsey, Henry Newell***
(Born: 10-02-1817 / Died: 27-06-1885) 125

G-5 ***Dr. Gururaju, M.***
(Born: 1897 / Died: 25-11-1963) 126

Dr. Nilmani Ghatak

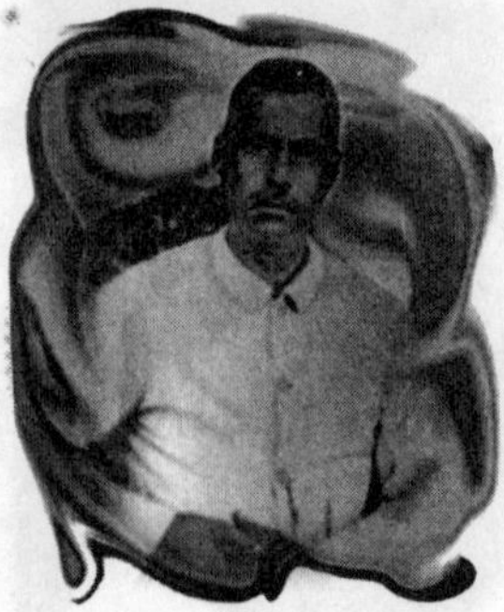

Born : 1872

Died : 19-01-1940

DEMISE

He was suffering from a dropsical condition, his activities were greatly reduced, the seriousness of his condition was not realised by many.

At age of 68 years he breathed his last on friday, 19th January, 1940 at 6 a.m. in Calcutta.

BIRTH

He was born in Gantikotulpore, a village in Bankura district of West Bengal.

EDUCATION

He passed the entrance examination of the university of Calcutta from Kotalpore English High School and for a meritorious result was Government scholarship of Rupees twenty per month. From Central College of Calcutta he passed B. A. examination with credit and distinction. He served as Head Master in several English High School but providence had something different for him.

CONVERSION TO HOMOEOPATHY

He was married in a very young age immediately after his graduation. His wife started suffering from a severe colick.

One night when his wife was in great distress he went to an allopathic physician for his wife's treatment but the physician refused to attend her at such large hours of the night. Their refusal was a turning point in his life and calder. The next morning he went to an ayurvedic physician and started visiting him regularly and associating with him closely, very soon he was taken in a disciple and later was able to cure his wife by his own treatment.

While he was serving as a Head Master of the Khanakul Krishna Nagar School, his eldest son was beised with an attack of cholera. A local ayurvedic physician was consulted but his treatment proved to be of no help and equally ineffective was allopathic treatment. The condition of the child deteriorated further. As a last resort a local homoeopath was called in and he cured the child. Ghatak's intelligence and magnisitive mind was soon attracted to homoeopathic literature. He was convinced of its logic and Superiority as a system of treatment.

At this time he passed the Bachelor of Law examination and joined the legal profession at Purulia. In his bisure times he used to practice homoeopathy. His fame reached great heights after he cured the daughter of the judge of Purulia.

His colleagues of legal profession conspired against him and filed a false case against him. Though he won the case but left Purulia. He went to Dhanbad and joined the legal profession there. His homoeopathic practice grew wider and wider and he was appointed as the RAJ PHYSICIAN of the Raja of Jharia. While he was in Shanbad his books "Chornic biseases And Their Treatment" and "Treatment of Malarial Fever" were published in Bangla.

Many of his articles published in the renowned journals Bangla monthly homoeopathic journal and Hahnemann Gleaning of Biff. (published by M/s Hahnemann Publishing Co.) and were widely read and appreciated.

He shifted to Calcutta and rented a house in Beadon Street and started his homoeopathic clinic there and after a short time he changed his residence to Bow Bazar Street and remained there till his last days.

Babu Prafulla Chandra Bhar always inspired him to write books on homoeopathy, after he has settled in Calcutta.

When the English monthly journal THE HANEMANNIAN GLEANINGS was started by M/s Hahnemann Publishing Co. in 1929 he was appointed as its Editor and he did his duties, as an editor, with great efficiency. He lift the editorship of this journal and started his own journal by the name MEDICAL ADVANCE.

PROFESSIONAL ACTIVITIES

He was a member of the international Hahnemannian Association of U.S.A.

He was elected as President of homoeopathic conferences held in Madras, Bombay and Calcutta.

HIS CHARACTER

He was very kind and always came forward to help the needy. He used to help many organisations financially.

Dr. Ghosh says of him "Intellectually sharp as a blade, socially meek as a lamb and professionally successful in his treatment, Dr. Ghatak was loved and revered by all who had occasion to come in close contact with him."

DEMISE

His second son, a homoeopath and Dr. Ghatak's assistant, expired and this loss probably hastened Dr. Ghatak's end.

Dr. S.C. Ghosh

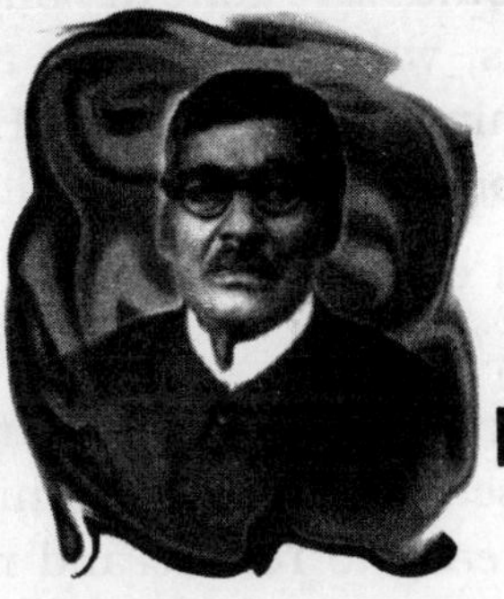

Born : 1870 **Died : 1953**

Hahnemann's homoeopathy, after its beginning in a small town, has in the last one and a half century completed a long journey, has faced rough weathers, many fire opponents, many hostile administrations, inimical rulers and political philosophies. It has lost many battles, but has won many wars, has lost few zealots and advocates, but gained many admirers and supporters. Seldom has its beginning, progress and development been free from biased rulings, personal vendates and at times singular persecutions. No other Medical Science has suffered such unkind fate and such brute opposition, of hundreds of opposition and opression.

The story of its progress and propagation is glorified by individual courage, sacrifice and determination. It is the fascinating story of resentment of fanatic medical and administrative Louise XVIII (Sixteenth) in different countries is speaking in different languages and practice in different cultures. The ability to tell this story has been possessed six very few and that is why Bradford, Kleinert Rapou, Richard Haehl, Ameke, King, Tischner, Ruthven Mitchel, Harris L. Coulter have immortalize themselves. They had one quality of objective perception and the truthful narration.

India the largest country where homoeopathy has taken its last shelter has the largest number of homoeopathic practitioners, examining universities, registering board and teaching institutions. But it has one and only one historian.

So on the rain-wet morning on the 8th of August, 1953, in the death of Dr. S.C. Ghosh India lost its Bradford, and Stonehome, its Kleinert and Ameke, its Mitchel and Rapou.

Had it not been for the individual effort and personal pen of Dr.

S.C. Ghosh the umbilical cord linking the present homoeopathy with its past pioneers would have gone dry and would have remained unborn whatever books, write-up articles and other publications have appeared concerning the history of Homoeopathy these all have been copy and reproduction of the writing of Dr. Ghosh.

On the other hand equally great were his contributions as a prover of homoeopathic drugs.

Today after four decades of his departure from this planet it is difficult to correctly assess the reasons of his interest in history of homoeopathy but it is easy to realize and perceive the necessity, importance and perfection of his work. Greater realization of the difficulties in compiling the history of homoeopathy has added greater reverence and sharper focus to Dr. S.C. Ghosh and his works.

FAMILY AND ANCESTORS

His ancestors belonged to the Jessore district of East Bengal now known as Bangladesh.

BIRTH

Dr. S.C. Ghosh was born on the 24th of July, 1870 at Jessore in East Bengal, now known as Bangladesh.

PROFESSIONAL ATTACHMENTS

1949 : On 5th December elected as a "Corresponding Member" of The foundation for Homoeopathic Research Incorporation, New York.

1931 : Elected President of the First All Bengal & Assam Homoeopathic Conference at Calcutta.

1933 : Re-elected President of the 2nd All Bengal & Assam Homoeopathic Conference at Tangail, Maimansing.

President of the All India Homoeopathic Conference at Gaya.

HIS SERVICES

He was instrumental in the inception and establishment of General Council and State faculty of Homoeopathy Medicine, Bengal.

Section-G : Dr. Ghosh, S.C.

HIS PROFESSIONAL CAREER

In the early part of 1903 he came from Midnapur and settled down at Bhawanipur. He started Homoeopathic practice in Midnapur, West Bengal from 1898.

HIS CONTRIBUTIONS

Many of his articles were published in the Homoeopathic World and B.H. Journals of Britain, Homoeopathic Recorder, Hahnemannian Monthly, North American Journal of Homoeopathic Progress, Cleveland's Medical and Surgical Reports, Medical Advance of U.S.A., Review Homoeopathic Francaise of France, Allegeimine Homoeoapthische Zeitung.

1900 : His paper on "Plague and Diabetes Mellitus" were accepted by 6th Ouin-quiennal International Homoeopathic Congress, in July at Paris, in 1900, and published in their transaction.

1911 : His writing "Beriberi and Justicia Adhatoda" was accepted by 8th Homoeopathic Congress of 1911 at London and published in their transaction.

1927 : His writing "Tuberculinum and Pneumonia" was printed in the transaction of the 9th International Homoeopathic Congress, London. Cholera and its homoeopathic treatment.

1935 : Life of Dr. Mahendra Lal Sircar, (2nd edition) Bisuchika Darpan (Bangla).

HOMOEOPATHIC MATERIA MEDICA (BANGLA) WORKER

He proved Ficus Relgiosa (Aswatha), Nyctanthes arbortristis (Shephalica), Justicia adhatoda (Basaka), and these drugs were included in Materia Medica of J.H. Clarke., W. Boerick, Blackwood. He was a corresponding member of :

1. American Institute of Homoeopathy.
2. British Homoeopathic Medical Society.
3. Hahnemann Institute of Brazil.
4. Homoeopathic Medical Academy of Barcelona.
5. American Association of Clinical Research.
6. California State Homoeopathic Medical Society.

HONORARY MEMBER OF

1. International Hahnemannian Association of America.
2. Liga Hispana Americana Homoeopathica of Barcelona, and
3. New Health Society of London.

HE WAS ELECTED AS

1. One of the Vice Presidents of the International Homoeopathic Congress, London, 1927.

LITERARY CONTRIBUTION

He was editor-in-chief of *Hahnemannian Gleanings* from 1932 to 1953 and chief editor of *Hahnemann (Bengalee)*. He worked as an associate editor of *Pacific Coast Journal of Homoeopathy*.

DEMISE

Although 84 years old he was keeping a good health. But suffered an attack of apoplexy at about 11 A.M. on the 5th of August and the morning of 8th August 1953 ended the life of Dr. Ghosh who has given great, valuable service to homoeopathy.

DESCENDANTS

Dr. Ghosh was survived by his son Dr. S.K. Ghosh, who is a practicing homoeopath, unasuming, honest and sincere to his job and patients.

His Grandson, a highly qualified engineer, is employee on a high post in U.S.A.

Thus the family link of Dr. S. C. Ghosh with homoeopathy ends with his son Dr. S.K. Ghosh.

WRITINGS OF DR. S.C. GHOSH

1935 : Treatment of every type of cough in Homoeopathic System (Bangla). Reference Hahnemann, Jaistha, 1342, P. 12.

: Continuation.
Reference Hahnemann, Sraban, 1342, P. 120.

: Continuation.
Reference Hahnemann, Asar, 1342, P. 57.

: Continuation.
Reference Hahnemann, Aswing, 1342, P. 225.

: Continuation.
Reference Hahnemann, Kartik, 1342, P. 318.

: Continuation.
Reference Hahnemann, Magh, 1342, P. 468.

: Symphoricarpus racimosa (Bangla)
Reference Hahnemann, Paus, 1342, P. 393.

: Sulphur and its practical hints (Bangla).
Reference Hahnemann, Phalgun, 1342, P. 505.

: Encephalitis Lethargica : My Experience and its Homoeopathic treatment. (Bangla)
Reference Hahnemann, Phalgun, 1342, P. 545.

: Sulphur and its practical hints (Continuation) (Bangla).
Reference Hahnemann, Chaitra, 1342, P. 567.

1936 : Calcarea carb (Bangla).
Reference Hahnemann. Baisakh, 1343, P. 640.

1937 : Poetry on Hahnemann, (Bangla)
Reference Hahnemann, Jaistha, 1343, P. 1.

: Diphtheria (Bangla).
Reference Hahnemann, Jaistha, 1343, P. 36.

: Continuation.
Reference Hahnemann, Sraban, 1343, P. 142.

: Continuation.
Reference Hahnemann, Kartik, 1343, P. 361.

: My Experience.
Reference Hahnemann, Agrahan, 1343, P. 281.

: Tabacum (Bangla).
Reference Hahnemann. Magh, 1343, P. 449.

: Sepia (Bangla).
Reference Hahnemann, Phalgun, 1343, P. 525.

: Indication for application of some medicine (Bangla).
Reference Hahnemann. Chaitra, 1343, P. 594.

: Effect of Homoeopathic Medicine in tuberculosis (Bangla).
Reference Hahnemann. Chaitra, 1343, P. 604.

1938 : Urtica urens, My Experience (Bangla).
Reference Hahnemann, Baisakh, 1344, P. 636.

: Cephalandra indica (Bangla).
Reference Hahnemann. Asar, 1344, P. 57.

: Phaseolus nanus (Bangla).
Reference Hahnemann. Sraban, 1344, P. 137.

: Ignatia (Bangala)
Reference Hahnemann, Bhadra, 1344, P. 195.

: Antimonium oxidatum, My Experience (Bangla).
Reference Hahnemann, Aswin, 1344, P. 230.

: Vesicaria Communis, My Experience (Bengali).
Reference Hahnemann, Kartik, 1344, P. 281.

: Role of Radium bromide in the world of Homoeopathic Treatment. (Bangla).
Reference Hahnemann, Agrahan, 1344.

: Ferrum phosphoricum (Bangla).
Reference Hahnemann, Paus, 1344, P. 393.

: Address to the All Orissa Homoeopathic Congress (Bangla).
Reference Hahnemann, Magh, 1344, P. 485.

: Continuation.
Reference Hahnemann, Phalgun, 1344, P. 527.

: Clinical Picture of some Homoeopathic Medcine, (Bangla).
Reference Hahnemann, Chaitra, 1344, P. 582.

1938 : My Experience in treatment of Appendicitis (Bangla).
Reference Hahnemann, Asar, 1345, P. 108.

: Sanguinaria canadensis, My Experience (Bangla).
Reference Hahnemann, Sraban, 1345, P. 168.

: Some new facts on Lycopodium (Bangla).
Reference Hahnemann, Bhadra, 1345, P. 257.

: Homoeopathic treatment of influenza (Bangla).
Reference Hahnemann, Aswin, 1345, P. 257.

: Continuation.
Reference Hahnemann, Kartik, 1345, P. 321.

: Continuation.
Reference Hahnemann, Agrahan, 1345, P. 385.

:	Discussion, Pulsatilla and Kalium sulph (Bangla). Reference Hahnemann, Magh, 1345, P. 513.
:	Hypericum perforatum, My Opinion (Bangla). Reference M. Hahnemann, Phalgun, 1345, P. 577.
:	Comparison and differentiation between Sepia, Natrium muriaticum and Phosphorus. (Bangla). Reference Hahnemann, Chaitra, 1345, P. 684.
1939 :	Hahnemann (Bangla Poetry). Reference Hahnemann, Jaistha, 1346. P. 1.
:	Life of Dr. Rajendra Lal Dutta (Bangla). Reference Hahnemann, Jaistha, 1346. P. 11.
:	Life history of Dr. Mahendra Lal Sircar (Bangla). Reference Hahnemann, Asar, 1346, P. 64.
:	Continuation. Reference Hahnemann, Sraban 1346. P. 129.
:	Dr. T. Berini (Bangla). Reference Hahnemaan, Bhadra, 1346. P. 193.
:	Efficacy of Lachesis (Bangla). Reference Hahnemann, Bhadra, 1346, P. 249.
:	Role of Cephalandra indica in Blood Sugar and Diabetes (Bangla). Reference Hahnemann, Aswin, 1346, P. 257.
:	Life of Dr. C. F. Tonneer (Bangla). Reference Hahnemann, Aswin, 1346, P. 261.
:	Solidago verger in Cystitis (Bangla). Reference Hahnemann, Agrahan, 1346, P. 438.
:	Life of Dr. L. Salger, (Bangla). Reference Hahnemann, Kartik, 1346, P. 321.
:	Life of Dr. Behari Lal Bhaduri (Bangla). Reference Hahnemann, Agrahan, 1346, P. 385.
:	Life of Dr. D. N. Roy (Bangla). Reference Hahnemann, Paus, 1346, P. 449.
:	Continuation. Reference Hahnemann, Magh, 1346, P. 513.
:	Cont. of Life of Dr. Lokenath Maitra (Bangla). Reference Hahnemann, Chaitra, 1346, P. 641.

: Life of Dr. Lokenath Maitra (Bangla).
Reference Hahnemann, Phalgun, 1346, P. 577.

1940 : Cont. of Life of Dr. Loke Nath Maitra, (Bangla).
Reference Hahnemann, Baisakh, 1347, P. 707.

: Life of Dr. T. Berigny (English).
Reference The Hanemannian Gleaning, April, P. 113.

: Life of Dr. Leopold Salzer (English).
Reference The Hanemannian Gleanings, November, P. 505.

: Comparison and differentiation between Sepia, Natrium muriaticum, and Phosphorus (Bangla).
Reference Hahnemann, Chaitra, 1345, P. 705.

: Life of Dr. D. N. Roy (Bangla).
Reference Hahnemann, Magh, 1346, P. 513.

: Life of Dr. Loknath Maitra (Bangla).
Reference Hahnemann, Phalgun, 1346. P. 577.

: Role of Arnica montana in Cancer. (Bangla).
Reference Hahnemann, Phalgun, 1346. P. 589.

: Life of Dr. Loknath Maitra (Cont). Bengali.
Reference Hahnemann, Chaitra, 1346. P. 641.

: Continuation.
Reference Hahnemann, Baisakh, 1347, P. 707.

: Life of Dr. Mahendra Lall Sircar (English).
Reference The Hahnemannian Gleanings, February, P. 3.

: Continuation.
Reference The Hahnemannian Gleanings, March, P. 87.

: Life of Dr. T. Berigny (English).
Reference The Hahnemannian Gleanings, April, P. 113.

: Cont. of Life of Dr. Lokenath Maitra (English).
Reference The Hahnemannian Gleaning, September, P. 393.

: Life of Dr. Leopold Salzar (English).
Reference The Hahnemannian Gleanings, November, P. 505.

Section-G : Dr. Ghosh, S.C.

1941 : Life of Dr. C. F. Tonneere (English)
Reference The Hahnemannian Gleanings, November.

: Life of Dr. Jagat Chandra Roy (English).
Reference The Hahnemannian Gleanings, July.

: Life of Dr. John Martin Honigberger (Bangla).
Reference Hahnemann, Jaistha, 1347, P. 4.

: Life of Dr. Bama Charan Das (Bangla).
Reference Hahnemann, Pholgun, 1347, P. 577.

: Life of Dr. Akshoy Dutta (Bangla).
Reference Hahnemann, Chaitra, 1347, P. 193.

: Life of Dr. Jaggat Chandra Roy (Bangla).
Reference Hahnemann, Chaitra, 1347. P. 641.

: Life of Dr. M. M. Basu (Bangla).
Reference Hahnemann, Chaitra, 1347, P. 65.

: Life of Dr. Brajendra Nath Bondopadhya (Bangla).
Reference Hahnemann, Sraban, 1347, P. 129.

: Dr. Nagendra Nath Majumdar (English).
Reference The Hahnemannian Gleanings. September.

: Myristica sebifera (Bangla).
Reference Hahnemann, Jaistha, 1347. P. 9.

: Iris versicolor (Bangla).
Reference Hahnemann, Jaistha, 1347, P. 73.

: Efficacy of Natrium muriaticum in continuous Malaria fever (Bangla).
Reference Hahnemann, Aswin, 1347, P. 264.

: Gymnema sylvestre (Bangla).
Reference Hahnemann, Sraban, 1347, P. 144.

: Homoeopathy in treatment of Append-icitis (Bangla).
Reference Hahnemann, Aswin, 1347, P. 315.

: Life of Dr. Nagendra Nath Majumdar (Bangla).
Reference Hahnemann, Magh, 1347, P. 513.

1942 : Life of Dr. C. F. Tonneer (Bangla).

: Life of Dr. Kishori Mohan Bandopadhya (Bangla).
Reference Hahnemann, Baisakh, 1348, P. 725.

: Case History of Some treated patients (Bangla).
Reference Hahnemann, Agrahan, 1348, P. 436.

: Lathyrus : My Experience (Bangla).
Reference Hahnemann, Phalgun, 1348, P. 588.

: My Experience of Arsenicum iodatum and Ceanothus or Chionauthus in Malaria fever with enlarged spleen and liver (Bangla).
Reference Hahnemann, Chaitra, 1348, P. 653.

1943 : History of Homoeopathy in India (English).

1944 : Chionanthus virginica (Bangla).
Reference Hahnemann, Bhadra, 1350. P. 145.

: In the memory of Hahnemann (Bangla Poetry).
Reference Hahnemann, Jaistha, 1350, P. 1.

: Achyranthes aspera : My Experience. (Bangla).
Reference Hahnemann, Sraban, 1349, P. 129.

: Efficacy of Atista indica in cure of intermittant fever (Bangla).
Reference Hahnemann, Asar, 1349, P. 65.

: Coleus aromaticus : My Experience (Bangla).
Reference Hahnemann, Bhadra, 1349, P. 193.

: Luffa amara : My Experience (Bangla).
Reference Hahnemann, Aswin, 1349, P. 256.

: Treatment of Bacillary Dysentry: My Experience (Bangla).
Reference Hahnemann, Magh, 1349, P. 513.

: Carbo vegetabilis in treatment of Cholera with blood vomiting (Bangla).
Reference Hahnemann, Phalgun, 1349, P. 578.

: Tabacum: My Experience (Bangla).
Reference Hahnemann, Chaitra, 1349, P. 633.

: Application of Tuberculium in Pneumonia; My Experience (Bangla).
Reference Hahnemann. Baisakh, 1349.

1944 : Alfalfa : My Experience (Bangla).
Reference Hahnemann, Baisakh, 1350, P. 694.

1945 : In the memory of Hahnemann (Bangla).
Reference Hahnemann. Jaistha, 1351, P. 1.

: Autobiography of a Herb (Bangla).
Reference Hahnemann, Sraban, 1351, P. 118.

	:	Antobiography of a Herb (Bangla). Reference Hahnemann, Aswin, 1351, P. 200.
1946	:	Hahnemann ((Bangla Poetry). Reference Hahnemann, Jaistha, 1353, P. 1.
1951	:	Present Position of Homoeopathy in the United States of America (English). Reference The Hahnemannian Gleanings, August. P. 275.
	:	Reply to the letters of Dr. G. Dirghangi & Dr. C. M. Bhatia of Calcutta (English). Reference The Hahnemannian Gleanings, October, P. 364.

Dr. Gustav Wilhelm Gross

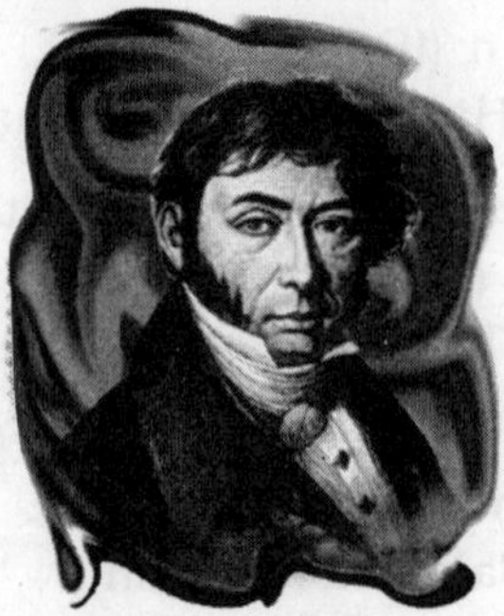

Born : 06-09-1794 **Died : 18-09-1847**

Gustav Wilhelm Gross was one of the earliest disciples of Hahnemann who remained faithful and devoted, till last, to him and his system of healing. He had viewed from very close range the infancy of homoeopathy, had grown with it and had observed many of the effects of many medicines upon himself and others and was blessed with Hahnemann's personal guidance. All of these helped him to develop a keen aptitude for practical side of the art of healing, so as to become the successful physician that he was, in the true sense of the word.

ANCESTORS & FAMILY

Mr. Johann Gottfried Gross was a pastor. His wife, Christiane Eleonore, was born at Schuricht. They had eight children.

BIRTH

Gustav Wilhelm Gross was the eldest son of the eight children of Gottfried Gross and Christiane Eleonore. He was born on the 6th of September, 1794 at Kaltenborn near Jueterbogk.

EDUCATION

He received his early education from his father and in 1809 was sent to the Gymnasium (Grammar School) at Naumburg on the Saale. He wanted to be a pastor and distinguished himself in the study of ancient languages especially Latin and Hebrew. He stayed there until the autumn of 1814 and then went to Leipzig to study medicine. He suffered in childhood from skin diseases and it affected his health immensely. In 1815 he consulted Hahnemann and thus came in close contact with Hahnemann and then his career took a definite turn. He became a member of Hahnemann's proving group and made first experience with *Chamomilla.* Under Hahnemann's personal guidance and by his devotion he acquired exceptional knowledge of remedies such as few homoeopathic physicians possessed. He was taciturn and, at times, harsh in his social behaviour and always went his own straight way.

On the 6th of January, 1817 he graduated from the University of Halle, with a thesis titled "DISSERTATIO INAUGURALIS MEDICA, QUAE VERSATUR IN QUESTIONE: NUM USUI SIT IN CURATIONE MORBORUM NOMENCLATURA. He started homoeopathic practice at his place of birth, Kaltenborn, which in the meanwhile went under the administration of Prussia. Under the existing Prussian Medical law he had to undergo the Prescribed State Examination in the winter of 1817-18. This was a period of extreme financial difficulties for Gross who had limited means of earning and was compelled to proceed with his studies and his work in an artisan's house, in which he lived with his family under much hardship. In 1818 he received his final degree and settled in medical practice at the small town of Juterbogk, a provincial town situated near the Saxon frontier, upon the railroad between Leipzig to Berlin. The place and atmosphere suited his rugged nature. He declined offers to go to bigger towns like Magdeburg and Brunswick.

Inconveniences and hardships plagued him for many years. Homoeopathy was opposed by many persons especially medical men. His continued proving of drugs on himself, which he never concealed, led many people to believe that he was only experimenting with his patients.

But gradually and ultimately his reputation for brilliant cures and his writings became wide-spread and patients came to him even from Berlin and many consulted him by letters. The state authorities, in recognition to his talents and hard works, appointed him a member of the Supreme Examining Board for individual dispensing.

As in the professional life so in his personal life, sorrow was coupled with happiness. In 1818 he married Marianne Herrmann, the daughter of pastor Herrmann and he had five children but a promising son and beloved daughter died at young age.

HIS CONTRIBUTIONS

In 1822 his friend and first disciple of Hahnemann, Ernst Stapf founded the first homoeopathic journal, viz, ARCHIV FUR DIE HOMOEOPATHISCHE HEILKUNST and Dr. Gross became a devoted collaborator and began editing it from its 16th volume in 1837.

About 3000 patients were treated by him every year, which was supposed to be a very wide practice for a homoeopath in those days. He kept careful records and reports of each patient.

In 1832 another homoeopathic journal ALLGEMEINE HOMOEOPATHISCHE ZEITUNG was founded and Dr. Rummel was requested to take its charge. He would agree to it only on condition that Gross and Hartmann helped him and thus a wonderful team of homoeopathic journalists came to work together. Gross remained a co-editor of the journal upto 1845 (31st volume). This journal played a valuable role in the propagation and development of homoeopathy in its early history.

Gross introduced mineral waters in homoeopathic therapeutics. He wrote a book on *Teplitz* waters, made study of *Karlsbad* springs water and completed its pathogenesis of 185 symptoms in 1843.

Gross was the earliest pioneer who prepared and used high potencies and was severely criticised for it.

He was the first homoeopathic physician to make extensive studies in the application of homoeopathy in diseases of children and infants.

His value to homoeopathy and in the eyes of Hahnemann can be judged by a simple fact. In 1827 only he and Stapf were invited by Hahnemann to discuss the "Theory of Chronic Diseases" before its declaration to the world.

He assisted in translating the Materia Medica (1826-28) Pura in Latin.

Gross was involved in the proving of the following medicines: Aconitum napellus, Angustura vera, Acon., Angus., Argent, Arnica., Arsenicum album, Aurum, Belladonna, Can., Chel., China., Cocca, Dulc., Digit., Ac, Ferrum., Ignat., Mang., Maren., Moschus, Olean., Phos., Rheum, Ruta, Sambuc., Opium, Staph., Stan., Thuja, Verb.

HIS LITERARY CONTRIBUTIONS

His writings are distinguished by his calm sense of balance and serious scientific outlook. He hated fine flourishes of useless eloquence in writing.

The provings of many medicines on himself and the case history of his large number of patients are ample proof of his keenness in research. He contributed many highly praised essays. His criticism of Prof. Heinroth's ANTI ORGANON published as a supplement to the fifth volume of Organon in 1826 was a marvellous defence of homoeopathy. His reviews of many books were impassionate, scientific and respected.

He was elected as honorary member of The Silesian Union of Physicians, The Free Union of Leipzig and The Homoeopathic Societies of Paris, Palermo and Madrid.

HIS WRITINGS

1817 : His thesis for M.D. "Num usui sit in curatione morborum nomenclatura, Halle.

1820 : Remarks concerning The Hahnemannian System (Hufeland's journal).

1824 : Dietetic Guide for the Healthy and the Sick.

1826 : Homoeopathy Viewed in its Lights and Shadows. Critical Examination of the Anti-organon of Heinroth.

1829 : The Homoeopathic Science of Healing and its Relation to the State.

1831 : Concerning the mode of living of Parturient and lying-in-women and the Dietetic and Therapeutic treatment of the New born child.

: Cure of Cholera Merseburg.

1832 : The Mineral Springs at Teplits, with respect to their positive effects on Healthy men and as an Antipsoric remedy.

1833 : Concerning the treatment of the Mother and the Suckling from moment of conception.

1839-40 : Review of the History of Homoeopathy in the Last Decennium, with a Biograpahy of Muhlenbein, Leipzig.

1848 : Necessity for the Equalization of Homoeopathy with the older Medical School : A petition to the Ministry of Education. (It was a reprint from Allgemeine Homoeopathische Zeitung.)

1851 : Concerning the festival at the Unveiling of Hahnemann's Monument.

1851 : In addition to these he compiled two thick Volumes of Homoeopathic Repertory, each of about 1500 pages, which had additions by Hahnemann.

He was a co-editor of Allgemeine Homoeopathische Zeitung from 1832-1843.

During Hahnemann's Jubilee Celebration, he not only furnished most of the matter for the jubilee memorial but also elaborated most of it himself and then cheerfully handed it over to Rummel.

HIS CHARACTER

His appearance was almost angular and stiff and to strangers he appeared gruff and unapproachable. This impression was intensified by his somewhat bloated and bilious features.

His friends Rummel described him by saying, "He was earnest and truthful and one would rearly read his in-most thoughts. He won the full confidence of his patients, not by his outward appearance, but rather by his kindly nature and active benevolence."

But under this rough exterior he concealed a warm, tender heart. Rummel, his friend and another close associate of Hahnemann, wrote.

"Then I learned to appreciate more and more eminent worth of Gross as a man, friend and physician. His health was not materially affected at that time though he must have had to endure much hardship and excessive toil; but his features and the greenish gray colour of his somewhat puffed up cheeks, then already gave warning of the unseen enemy which was to end his busy life."

But inspite of his sickness and ill health he continued his practice and literary works. He was very easily inspired by new ideas and was so animated by new ideas that he used to grasp them with a fiery zeal and used to express them in a very impressive manner. This peculiarity in his character beguiled him into over hastiness and exaggeration, which he used to atone later for many sad hours and with bitter reproofs of his conscience. This nature in him led him once for a short sometime to the by-path of Isopathy. He was one of the early advocates of high potencies. He was bitterly criticised for this. He once prepared potencies with his own blood and used it in few cases for which he has been severely criticised by Dr. Baehm of German, Dr. Roth of France and Dr. Dudgeon of Britain.

After the death of his daughter under Hahnemann's treatment, he was frustrated and angry with Hahnemann and told Hahnemann that homoeopathy could not cure everything. Hahnemann was greatly displeased and accused him of vacillation and desertion. But at the time of Hahnemann's second marriage, he wrote a poem of fanatic jubilation and soon they became friends again. He was a great admirer of Mortiz Mueller and during Hahnemann's criticism of Dr. Mueller, Gross tried very hard to mediate between the two.

He was a simple man and liked to remain on his own. Although he was one of the original founders of the Central Association of Homoeopathy, he retired from its meetings in the later part of his life and declined the offer of chairmanship. He was happy in the company of Stapf and Rummel at Hahnemann's house in Koethen.

DEMISE

His liver trouble gave him more discomfort and very soon his trouble were complicated with gout, dropsy and lung trouble. He was not getting any relief from his own treatment or that of his friend Stapf or changes in Karlsbad and Baltic areas. He went for a recuperative change to his son-in-law Pastor Weise who had become a widower at Klebitz near Zahna and there, at the young age of 53 years, Dr. Gross breathed his last on the 18th of September, 1847. On 16th of September he told his closest friend Stapf, "I now have no more hope on earth, the account is closed, my path now tends upwards. He died in his sleep two days later. He was survived by his wife, a daughter and two sons, one of whom became a homoeopathic physician, and other became a master builder.

Hartmann said, "Gross was the most skillful prover of us all, and the symptoms observed by him have a great practical value. Indeed I place him with Franz and Stapf on an equality with Hahnemann." British Journal of Homoeopathy (Volume VI) described him as being perpetually occupied in the proving of which we owe entirely to him and most of those given us by Hahnemann being enriched by his experiments on himself and others.

Rapou, the French historian of homoeopathy, wrote, "He came little after Stapf and is after him the eldest of homoeopathic physicians. These two men adhered more strictly to the opinions and principles of homoeopathy than did many others."

Hartmann went further to say, "Time has shown that Hahnemann justly considered him one of his best pupils, for Gross was, in truth, during the whole course of his practice, the most zealous homoeopathist possible."

We have always known that "when the sifting hand of time

shall have winnowed the good seed from the chaff the name of Gross will be regarded and respected as one of the largest contributions to our remedial treasury."

SOURCE MATERIALS

Stapf. E. : Archiv Fur Die Homoeopathische Heilkunst, Volume XXII, Part-3.

Rummel : Allgemeine Homoeopathische Zeitung, Volume XXXIV, P. 193.

Bradford, T.L. : The Pioneer Practitioners of Homoeopathy, P. 20.

Haehl, Richard : Hahnemann : Life & Work, Vol. I. P. 377.

British Journal of Homoeopathy, Volume 30, P. 73.

Kleinert : Geschichte der Homo. P. 99.

Dudgeon : Lectures on Homoeopathy. North Western Journal of Homoeopathy. Volume IV. P. 85.

Medical Counsellor : Volume XI, P. 239.

Allgemeine Homo. Zeitung, Volume XXXVIII, P. 50.

Archiv Fur Die Homoeopathische Heilkunst : Volume XIV, No. 2., P. 50.

British Journal of Homoeopathy, Volume VI, P. 137, P. 25.

British Journal of Homoeopathy, Volume V, P. 131.

British Journal of Homoeopathy, Volume XXXII, P. 455.

Rapou, Anguste: Histoire de la Doctrine Homoeopathique, Volume 2. P. 430-600.

Neues ARCHIV for Homoeopathische Heil Kemsrs Volume I, 3, P. 35, 1844.

Dr. Henry Newell Guernsey

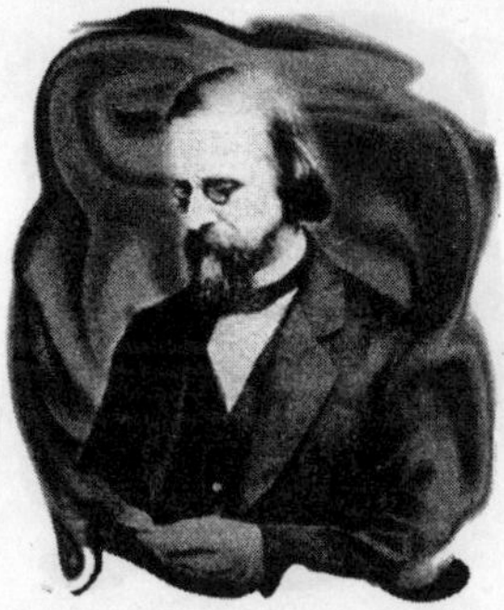

Born : 10-02-1817 **Died : 27-06-1885**

Henry Newell Guernsey, M.D., was born on the 10th of February, 1817 in Rochester, Vermont. In 1842 he received his medical degree from New York University. In 1856 he went to Philadelphia. He was professor of obstetrics at the new Homoeopathic Medical College. *He was an earnest, honest, and conscientious disciple of Hahnemann. He was renowned as a teacher of materia medica.*

He wrote the classic text : "The location of the Principles and Practice of Homoeopathy to Obstetrics and Disorders Peculiar to Women and Young Children."

He wrote the 'Keynote' method. He was the first public teacher of the 'Single Remedy' and the 'High Potency'.

In 1879, he was diagnosed with tuberculosis. Many people tried to prescribe for him but he always gave the same reply "I wish nothing 'but the simillimum in my case. As I have lined and practiced for others I will do by myself, for I know it is the right way. If I must die, I wish it recorded that I died true to my principles."

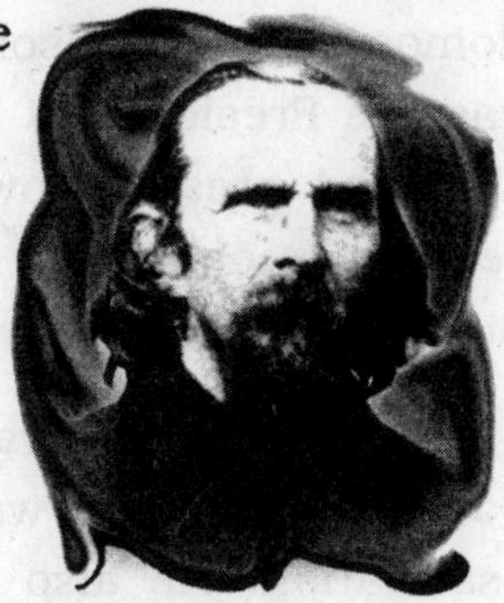

Dr. M. Gururaju

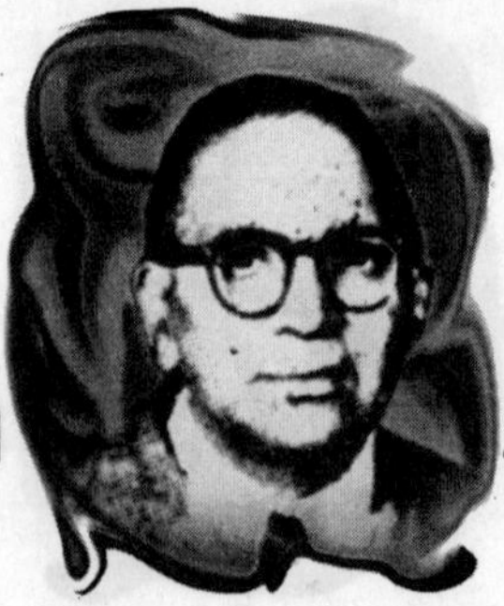

Born : 1897 Died : 25-11-1963

Dr. M. Gururaju was born near Gudivada, in June 1897. He first worked as a High School teacher; later he qualified himself as an L.M.P. from Stanely Medical School, Madras, in 1923. He set up practice at Gudivada in 1924 and was the first qualified allopathic practitioner in the taluk. He soon become popular as a very capable practitioner by and by the started taking part in the struggle for independence and went to jail in 1932. On his release from jail he discarded allopathy and started his newlife by starting as a homoeopathic practitioner.

He underwent postgraduate training in homoeopathy, in U.S.A. in 1936, under great stalwarts like Dr. Farrington, Dr. Spalding, Dr. Elizebeth Hubbard, and Dr. Woodbury. After returning from U.S.A., not satisfied with his own practice he tried to spread the system on scientific lines. With that idea, he started the 'Andhra Provincial Homoeopathic Medical College and Hospital' in 1945. He was a member of the State Homoeopathic Board and Homoeopathic Advisory Committee of the Government of India. He was the President of All India Institute of Homoeopathy in 1951-52, and presided over the All India Homoeopathic Conference, held at Lucknow in 1951. The College was recognized by the Government of Andhra Pradesh in 1958.

Dr. Gururaju was also elected to the Gudivada Municipal Council twice and was the President of the A.P. Homoeopathic Association. He also had the honour of being a member of the Expert Homoeopathic Committee, which was set up by the Andhra Pradesh Government in 1954 and a member of the Ad-hoc Syllabus

Committee and the Pharnacopoeia Committee in the Centre.

Dr. Gururaju brought his son Dr. Kutumba Rao, M.B.B.S., into the college in 1957. The college and hospital were mainly maintained by the main contribution of this single individual for a long time. The college got its own building in 1963. This noble soul, Dr. M. Gururaju, died on November 25, 1963. Later, the committee named the college after him. The college was handed over to the Government of Andhra Pradesh in 1968 and is now aptly called 'Dr Gururaju Government Homoeopathic Medical College.' The college is a living movement of his achievements and services.

Leadership is an opportunity to serve. It is not a trumpet call to self-importance.

SECTION-H .... Page 129 to 166

H-1 ***Dr. Hahnemann, Christian Friedrich Samuel***
(Born: 10-04-1755 / Died: 02-07-1843) 130

H-2 ***Dr. Hahnemann, Melanie d'Hervilly Gohier***
(Born: 02-02-1800 / Died: 27-05-1878) 139

H-3 ***Dr. Hartmann, Franz***
(Born: 18-05-1796 / Died: 10-10-1853) 141

H-4 ***Dr. Hazra, J.N.*** 145

H-5 ***Dr. Hempel, Charles Julius***
(Born: 05-09-1811 / Died: 24-09-1879) 146

H-6 ***Dr. Hering, Constantine***
(Born: 01-01-1800 / Died: 23-07-1880) 157

H-7 ***Dr. Honigberger, John Martin*** 161

H-8 ***Dr. Hughes, Richard***
(Born: 1836 / Died: 09-04-1902) 165

Dr. Christian Friedrich Samuel Hahnemann

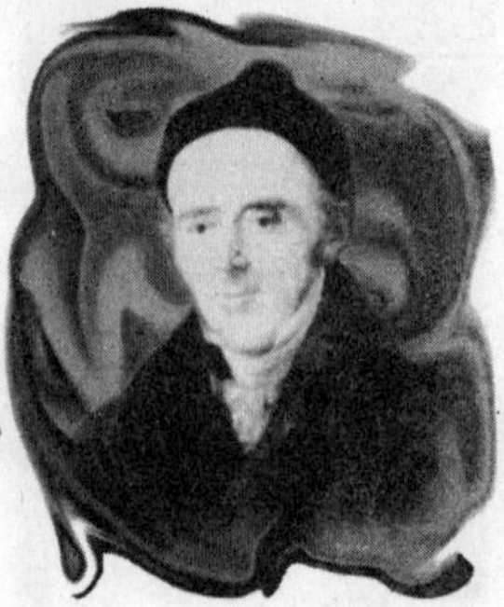

Born : 10-04-1755 **Died : 02-07-1843**

In the middle of the eighteenth century Germany consisted of the kings of Austria and Prussia, The Electors of Hanover and Saxony, 94 Spiritual and Lay Princes, 103 Counts, 40 Prelates, 53 Free towns, in all 30 separate territories.

Saxony in 1755, the year of the birth of Samuel Hahnemann, belonged to a loose confederation of German states. The most noteworthy feature of the period, before Hahnemann's birth, was the utter and complete exhaustion of the whole of the Germany as the result of the Thirty years' religious war of the previous century. Never was a country so scourged or so devastated.

ANCESTORS & FAMILY

Christoph Hahnemann, the painter, was the grand father of Samuel Hahnemann. He had seven children, three sons and four daughters. He was a prominent citizen of the summer resort town of Merseburg. His second son and fifth child born on 24th July, 1720 was Christian Gottfried Hahnemann. Christian Gottfried Hahnemann left Merseburg and settled in Meissen.

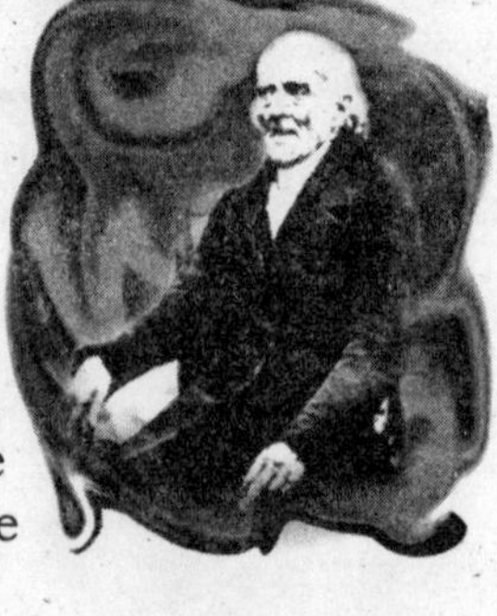

He married at the age of 28 years, on 27th November, 1748. His wife died after nine months giving birth to twins, one of whom was a still birth and another died after nine months. On the 2nd of November, 1750, he married Johanna Christiana Spiess, the only daughter of a captain and quarter master, on 6th of April, 1753. Gottfried acquired a house for himself. It was a corner house at the junction of two streets, the Newmarket and the Fleischsteg and hence it was called "the corner house."

BIRTH (11-04-1755)

Hahnemann was born in the early hours of Friday, the 11th April, 1755 and named Christian Frederick Samuel. This was recorded in the church register of Frauen-kirche in Meissen and has been corroborated by all the biographers of Hahnemann. But hahnemann in his autobiography, wrote "I was born on April 10th, 1755." Thus his birthday is observed and celebrated on 10th of April. Christian Gottfried Hahnemann lived and worked in a porcelain factory, named Meissen Pottery. Meissen was located on the banks of a small river called Meissen, near its junction with a larger river, Elbe. The town of Meissen was about twelve miles north-west of the city of Dresden.

EDUCATION (1755 TO 1779)

His father Gottfried and mother Johanna Christiana, taught him how to read and write. He was admitted to the Town School on the 20th of July, 1767. Several years of his childhood were spent in the Town School of Meissen and when of 12 years in age he was authorised to teach the rudiments of the Greek language to other students of the school. His father sent him as an apprentice to a grocery store in Leipzig so that the young boy may acquire the capacity to earn as soon as possible, but magister Mueller, the head of the Town School and some other teachers urged Gottfried Hanemann to allow his son Samuel to return to the school for tuition without usual fees. On 21st of November, 1770 Samuel went to the Prince's School. During school leaving ceremony at Prince's school Hahnemann composed and delivered, as was the custom, a Latin Oration titled, *THE WONDERFUL CONSTRUCTION OF THE HUMAN HAND.*

In 1775 he left for Leipzig with a total amount of 20-thalers for his support and this was the last money that he received from his father. In Leipzig he earned his bread by teaching German and French to a wealthy young Greek from Jassy in Moldavia. At the young age of Twenty-two he was well versed in Greek, Latin, English, Italian, Hebrew, Syriac, Arabic, Spanish, German and a little bit of Chaldiac and so translation of books was another means of earning his livelihood.

During his two-years' stay in Leipzig he translated John Stedman's *PHYSIOLOGICAL EXPERIMENTS AND OBSERVATIONS*

WITH COPPER, NUGENT'S ON HYDROPHOBIA, FALKONER'S ON MINERAL WATERS AND WARM BATH (2 Volumes). At that time, Leipzig had no hospital and so Hahnemann left for Vienna where he entered the hospital of the 'Brothers of Mercy, and was a favourite student of Dr. Von Quarin, Physician In-ordinary to the Empress Marie Theresa. Many years after, Hahnemann wrote, "I am indebted for my medical instinct to the practical genius of Dr. Quarin. I was the only one at that time whom he allowed to accompany him to his private patients."

While he was preparing to appear for his final examinations, Hahnemann's hard-earned savings were stolen away by one of his acquaintances. He was in acute financial hardship. The Governor of Transylvania, Baron Von Bruckenthal, invited him on honourable terms to go to Hermannstadt with him as his family physician and the custodian of his vast and important library. Thus Hahnemann got an opportunity of acquiring knowledge of some collateral sciences. After one year and nine months he went to Erlangen. He studied Botany under Royal Physician, Schreber. On the 10th April 1779, at the age of twenty-four years, Hahnemann obtained his degree, M.D., i.e. "DOCTOR OF MEDICINE" from Erlangen University. His thesis consisted of twenty printed pages on: *A CONSIDERATION OF THE ETIOLOGY AND THERAPEUTICS OF SPASMODIC AFFECTION.*

MEDICAL PRACTICE (1779-1792)

He began his practice in Hettstedt town. In the spring of 1731 he reached Dessau and at the end of the year he accepted the post of Medical Officer in Gommern, near Magdeburg.

His writings at this time were published in a journal named *"Kreb's Medical Observation."*

MARRIAGE

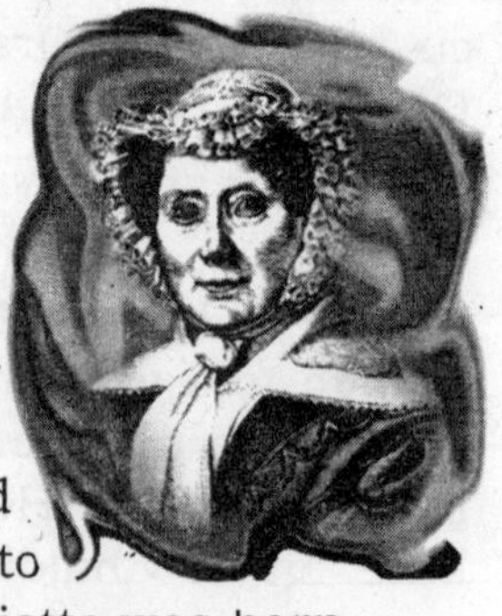

His interest and study of Chemistry brought him into contact with Haesler's Pharmacy, where he became acquainted with the later's stepdaughter Henriette Leopoldine Kuechler. Hahnemann married her on 17th November, 1782. The young doctor was aged 27 years and his bride was 9 years younger to him. In 1733, his first child, a daughter, Henriette was born.

Hannemann's translation of French Chemist J. Demachy's *"THE WHOLESALE MANUFACTURE OF CHEMICALS, OR THE*

Section-H : Dr. Hahnemann, C.F.S.

SCIENCE OF PREPARING CHEMICAL PRODUCTS IN FACTORIES" appeared in two volumes in 1785 with numerous footnotes, additional supplements, independent references, addenda, etc. During the year 1785-1789 this versatile author and translator published more than 2300 printed pages and from 1739 until the summer of 1792 his writings consisted of 4700 printed pages.

DISSATISFACTION WITH THE SYSTEM OF MEDICINE

His indignation and dissatisfaction with the medical practice of his time is best expressed in his own words in his essay *AESCULAPIUS IN BALANCE (1805).*

"Whoever expects from such processes that medicine will ever progress one step on the path to perfection has been denied by nature all the ability to distinguish probability form impossibility."

RICHARD HAEHL SAYS

"Hahnemann, the physician recognised more and more the complete insufficiency and unreliability of the science of his day. He withdrew more and more from medical practice. In 1793 he was mentioned in CRELL'S ANNAL (1, page 200) as "This famous analytical chemist."

In the spring of 1792 Hahnemann reached Gotha. In February 1796 issue of the DEUTSCHEN MONATSSCHRIFT, he emphasized the necessity of special attention of Psychiatry. The benevolent Prince Duke Ernst Won Sachsen-Gotha placed his hunting castle of Georgenthal at Hahnemann's disposal as a nursing home for mental patients. It was here that Klockenbring was brought as a patient and when he was cured the institution was closed in the summer of 1793.

DISCOVERY OF HOMOEOPATHY (1790-96)

In 1790 Hahnemann was translating, from English to German, **William Cullen's** *A TREATISE OF MATERIA MEDICA,* in two volumes of pages 468 and 672. Cullen had explained the malaria curing power of Cinchona to be due to its "tonic effect" on stomach. He challenged Cullen's contention of "Tonic effects on stomach by Cinchona bark" and to test the truth he started taking 4 drachms of Cinchona bark juice twice daily and the symptoms associated with intermittent fever appeared in him in succession. He suffered from malaria-like symptoms. It was here that Hahnemann sensed a law of cure. He understood that the effect that a substance produces on the healthy human body is the curative power by which it cures similar disease symptoms in sick persons.

Richard Haehl, wrote. "In Cullen's Materia Medica was established the first milestone on the new method of treatment of which Hahnemann was the originator."

From the years 1790 to 1805 his new system of treatment came slowly and gradually to a definite shape. Inspite of his constant change of places of residence (almost 7 times during this period), the hindrance of packing and unpacking, the difficulties of long journeys and the trill of setting in house, Hahnemann published over 5500 printed pages of original works, essays and translations, during this period of 15 years.

It was only 1796 that the *law of similars* became perfectly clear to Hahnemann and the new course was pointed out to the whole world in his essay, titled *"AN ESSAY ON A NEW PRINCIPLE FOR ASCERTAINING THE CURATIVE POWERS OF DRUGS AND SOME EXAMINATIONS OF THE PREVIOUS PRINCIPLES"*, published in *Hufeland's Journal* Volume II. parts 3 & 4, pages 391-439 and 465-561. He formulated his new discovery in these words.

"Every powerful medicinal substance produces in the human body a peculiar kind of disease the more powerful the medicine, the more peculiar, marked and violent the disease.

We should imitate nature which sometimes cures a chronic disease by super-adding another and employ in the (especially chronic) disease we wish to cure, that medicine which is able to produce another very similar artificial disease, and the former will be cured; similar similibus.

He put forward his new doctrine of *Similia Similibus Curantur (Like cures likes)* in contrast to the age old doctrine of *Contraria Contrariis Curantur (opposite cures opposites)*. "Thus 1796 is the year of birth of Homoeopathy", says Richard Haehl.

He called his system *Homoeopathy* in contrast to the prevailing system which he named *Allopathy.*

His eassy, *ARE THE OBSTACLES TO THE ATTAINMENT OF SIMPLICITY AND CERTAINTY IN PRACTICAL MEDICINE INSURMOUNTABLE?* was published in 1797 in *Hufeland's Journal*, Volume IV.

In 1806 he published his *Medicine of Experience* and in 1810 his *Organon Der Rationellen Helkunde* (Organon of the Rational Art of Healing) was published. In this book, he outlined and explained the concepts and methodology of homoeopathy and criticised other methods of treatment, especially allopathy.

OPPOSITION TO HOMOEOPATHY

T.L. Bradford, the immortal historian of homoeopathy said:

"The publication of this (Organon of Rational Art of Healing) was the signal for the commencement of a violent warfare against Hahnemann."

He was attacked in the medical journals, magazines, books and pamphlets were culminated against him and his doctrines. He was called "a charlatan, a quack, an ignoramus". In 1811 the first volume of his Materia Medica Pura, the record of symptoms produced by the drugs experienced on healthy human beings was published.

It is too ugly and too big a job to recite, yet too inhuman to forget the punitive treatment meted out to Hahnemann and his adherents by the profession and the state law of the time.

Bradford says: It is disgusting to state how it was received. It was and it remains forever, an inexcusable meanness of the whole profession."

Hahnemann was allowed to give lectures at Leipzig University. In the winter term of 1812 Hahnemann began his lectures, delivering them twice a week, on wednesday and saturdays from 2 to 3 p.m. About the attitude of the opponents of homoeopathy Hartmann wrote:

"Perpetual revelry from the students, poisonous looks from the most of the professors, anxious desire of everybody to avoid more intimate intercourse with us — as if we were infected with some pestilential eruption."

However, Hahnemann was able to gather his first band of dedicated disciples who remained faithful to him and homoeopathy till the end of their physical lives. He was able to form a group of his drug provers.

In 1816, Hahnemann, the medical logician, entered into a news paper feud with Dr. Dzondi of Halle who has been advocating the use of cold water as the only sure means of curing burns of every kind quickly and painlessly. Hahnemann had suggested "the preference of (warm) spirits of wine to cold water in severe burns." The dispute went on throughout the whole year of 1817 until November, 1818 without any positive result. Riding over the dispute came another two-pronged attack — one from Dr. J.K. Bischoff through his work (1819) entitled *"views on the methods of healing upto this time and on the first principles of the homoeopathic theory of disease"* and another from Professor Puchelt through his eassy in Hufeland's Journal, Part 6, 1819.

Prince Schwarzenberg who had been the General Officer Commanding of the Allied armies against Napoleon, was paralysed by a stroke on the 13th of January, 1817. The Prince came to Leipzig with a large retinue and two doctors to put himself under Hahnemann's treatment. He improved under homoeopathic treatment but he soon fell back to the old habit of strong drinks and started taking allopathic medicines and other measures from time to time.

That was five weeks before the prince's death and Hahnemann never visited him again. The prince died after six months of his arrival in Leipzic from another stroke on the 15th October 1820. Prince Schwazenberg's death brought intense agony to the Austrians and gave opportunity to allopaths for attacking homoeopathy and Hahnemann. It brought intensive and violent persecution to Hahnemann and his new system of healing. The Saxon Government which had withheld their judgement in the complaint filed by 'Apothecaries', an association of the pharmacists, against Hahnemann the royal decree of 30th November, 1820 almost prohibited him from dispensing his own medicines.

The *'Apothecaries' Guild* as a whole and its Leipzic branch were raising hue and cry against Hahnemann who was dispensing his own medicines and that too in small quantities. They had only a few years ago, acclaimed Hahnemann for his widely recognised book *Apothecaries Lexicon* which served as a practical book for pharmacists and compounders. A prevailing law "Constitutions Federici II Imperatories" ordered that the compounding of mixtures can be done only by the apothecaries and there were other laws and statues which prevented the physicians from giving any medicine directly to their patients. In 1819 they submitted a complaint to the Council of the Town of Leipzic accusing Hahnemann of violating the law. On the 9th of February, 1820 Hahnemann was brought before a court which ordered a penalty of 20 thalers.

Thirteen physicians of Leipsic published a long eassy in a news paper, viz., LEIPZIGER ZEITUNG, of 5th February, 1821, against Hahnemann. Some of the doctors and apothecaries attempted to drive Dr. Hahnemann by force out of Leipzic, however, Dr. Volkamann, the town clerk Dr. Linder and forty other citizen of Leipzig entered a signed protest against this high handedness and as a result Hahnemann was able to remain in Leipzic. In June,

Section-H : Dr. Hahnemann, C.F.S.

1821 he left for Koethen accompanied by Heynel and Mossdorf.

Hahnemann endured every hit of the madness with grace and determination. In the preface of the second edition of Organon of Medicine he wrote;

"Physicians are my brethren. I have nothing against them personally."

He further said, "I care nothing for the ingratitude and persecution which have pursued me on my wearisome pilgrimage. The great objects I have pursued have prevented my life from being joyless."

About his opponents he wrote "...... Rather compassionate the poor blind infatuated creatures, it is mortification enough for them to be unable to accomplish anything valuable."

And then the benevolence of Duke Ferdinand Anhalt-Koethen came to his rescue. The Duke invited Hahnemann to live and practice in Koethen, a country town of 6000 inhabitants, where he was subsequently elected as Privy Councillor.

In 1822, Stapf published the first periodical of homoeopathy, *The Archiv, for the Homoeopathic Science of Healing* with the help of Gross and Mueller. In 1828 Hahnemann's famous classic: *Chronic Diseases Their nature and Homoeopathic Cure* was published.

The jubilee of Hahnemann's Doctorate was celebrated by his students, disciples, admirers and followers of Europe on 10th of April 1829, and the *Society of homoeopathic Physicians of Leipzig* was founded. Hahnemann's wife Johanna Henriette, after near[ly] forty-eight years of a happily married life and the mother of h[is] eleven children, died on 31st of March, 1830.

For four years Hahnemann was cared and protected by his daughters and when smiles of the Goddess of fortune were all around him, cupid smiled again in his life.

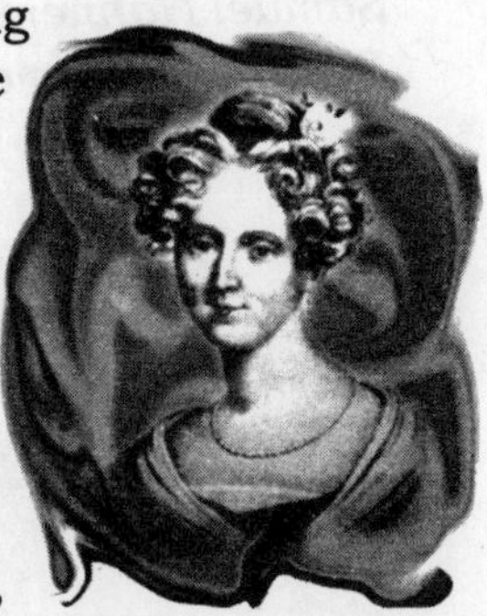

On the 8th of October 1834, a charming French lady, Marie Melanie De Hervilly came to consult him for her skin ailments. She was an artist and a poetess, rich and famous. The beauty was attracted to the genius and the genius to the talent. The differences in age stood as no bar. Hahnemann (aged 80 years) married for the second time on the new year day of 1835... and this time his bride (aged 35 years) was 45 years junior to him. Melanie, took Hanemann to France in June 1835. By a Royal decree of August 12th, 1835, Hahnemann was granted the right to practice homoeopathy in Paris. In France, Hahnemann received the reward of his years of trials and tribulations, hardships and hunger, struggles and starvations.

DEMISE

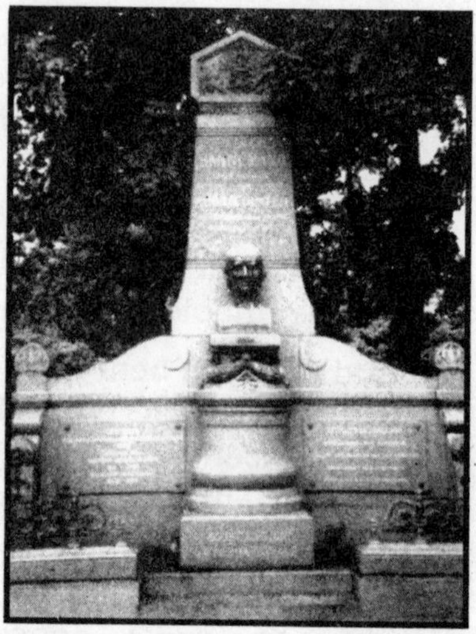

The great master breathed his last at 5 a.m. on the 2nd of July, 1843 at the age of 88 years 2 months 21 days and 3 hours.

Bradford described Hahnemann as:

"Scholar whom scholars honoured and respected; physiciar whom physicians feared; philologis with whom philologists dreaded t dispute; chemist who taugh chemists, philosopher whor adversity nor honour had power t change."

Hahnemann's befitting statues and monuments are in Pere La Chaise in Paris, in Koethen, in Leipzig and in Washington of U.S.A.

The inscription on his monument of the Pere La Chaise Cemetry of Paris says:

"Standing between the inorganic
And the Organic World
Uniting them for benefit of the sick;
Earning their gratitude.
Looking towards eternity
Samuel Hahnemann,
Benefactor of mankind,"

Dr. Melanie d'Hervilly Gohier Hahnemann

Born : 02-02-1800

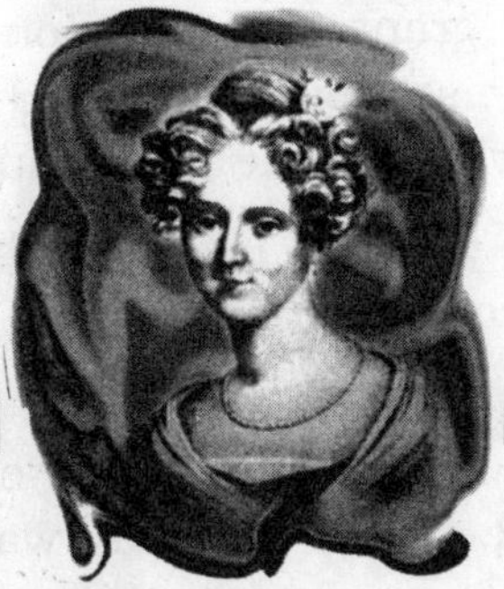

Died : 27-05-1878

On the 2nd of February, 1800 Melanie was born in Paris.

When she was 15 yrs. old her father sent her to line with the family of the painting teacher, Guillaume Guillon-Lethiere, because Melanie's relationship with his mother was not cordial. At the age of 20 she became a successful painter.

Melanie was also interested in the poetry, during the 1820's she wrote poetry and became involved with the complex politics of the Republican wing of French political life. She knew many of the poets and writers of that time. She wrote poetry to and for Louis Jerome Gohier, a well known political leader. Gohier was added to Melanie's name after gohier's death, who left both money and his name for her in 1830, so that his name would be spoken of with an esteem equal to hers.

In 1832, during the cholera epidemic, on seeing the success of Dr. Omin, who treated the victims of this epidemic with homoeopathy, melanie became interested in homoeopathy. With great efforts she found a copy of the 4th edition of the *Organon* and read it. She left for Kothen to meet Hahnemann, after 15 days journey she reached Kothen on October 7, 1834. She found the widowed Hahnemann living with his two daughters. Hahnemann proposed to Melanie within three days of their meeting.

At kothen, Melanie stayed with one of Hahnemann's friend. While in Kothen the painted, rode worse-back, practiced pistol-shooting, and hunted.

After receiving the permission from Melanie's father to wed,

Hahnemann and Melanic were married on January 18, 1835. As Melanie was a catholic, she learned the Lutheran creed to be married to Hahnemann. After living for a while in Kothen, the couple left for Paris on June 7. Hahnemann set up a busy practice in Paris when he was granted permission to practice medicine there. Melanie became his pupil and shared the practice with him. Often, she would prescribe and he would supervise.

Inspite of his busy practice Hahnemann enjoyed a social life and often went to the concerts or the opera with Melanie and her father.

When Hahnemann died Melanie lay next to his embalmed body for almost a week. Then, his body was placed in the small vault at Montmartre.

After Hahnemann's death Melanic continued to practice homoeopathy and in 1847, on the 20th of February she was brought to court for practicing without qualification. Melanie claimed for the right to practice homoeopathy because she had been granted a diploma from Allentown, Penneylvania in 1840. She was found guilty even after Dr. Crorerio, who supervised her cases, spoke on her behalf. She was fined 100 francs and told to cease practice.

In 1843, Melanie adopted a five year old girl, Sophie, shortly before Hahnemann's death. Ophie was the daughter of a patient and friend of Hahnemann, the musician Anton Bohrer. In 1857, Sophie was married to Karl Boenninghausen, the son of Clemens Maria Franz Von Boenninghausen. Melanie obtained the permission for Karl to practice medicine in Paris and again she started to practice under Karl's Supervision.

In 1871, Karl & Sophine left Paris and moved to Westphalia where Melanie would visit on occasion.

Melanie died in Paris, on the 27th of May, 1878.

Dr. Franz Hartmann

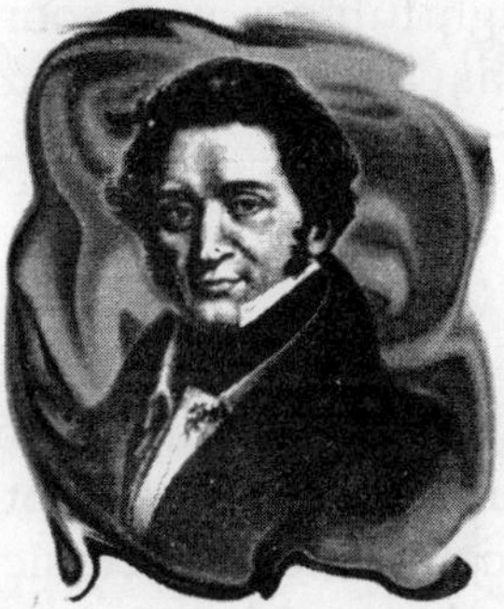

Born : 18-05-1796 **Died : 10-10-1853**

"Struggle" is the word which would describe Dr. Franz Hartmann's life in one world.

He came from a poor family. In his early life he has to struggle against poverty. In his academic life he has to bear the grudge of many for his fault of being an admirer of homoeopathy, in practice Hartmann has to struggle against the allopaths and even some homoeopaths and, last but not the least, he has to struggle through out his life history against his ill-health.

Franz Hartmann was born on 18th of May, 1976, the year of birth of Homoeopathy and the year in which the discovery of homoeopathy was made known to the whole world by its founder, Master Hahnemann. Rranz was born in Delitsch, the p;ace where his father worked as a school teacher.

As a young boy Franz was very keen and intgelligent though has a sickly appearance.

In 1810, at the early age of fourteen years, he was studing Theology in Grammar School of Chemnitz and also giving tutions to the children of poor weavers.

Soon Hartmann choose to become a physician and went to Leipsic in 1814 at the age of 18 years.

In Leipsic the met his former mate Christian Gottlob Karl Hornburg who had also left theology for medicine. They now were sharing the same room and very soon both were following the same principle in medicine. Hartmann was impressed by Hornburg who was a strong follower of Homoeopathy and Hahnemann. Through Hornburg he met Hahnemann. Hartmann was very much attracted by personality of the writing is a summarised version by Dr. Subhas singh from Dr. Mahendra Singh's writing presented at Indian Homoeopathic Medical Leagu. W. B. Semminar, May 1989. Hahnemann and his trughtfulness and soon became a member of **Prover's Union** and was a frequent visitor and well-known to Hahnemann's family circle.

MEDICAL EDUCATION

His homoeopathic activities earned for him the anger of allopaths. Thinkng that this may hinder his getting this degree, Hartmann after 2½ years. on 19th of September, 1817, went to Berlin. But very soon he came back to Leipsic at the commencement of long holidays because "he could there puruse his homoeopathic studies more zealously."

In March 21st, 1819 he received his medical diploma in Jena. It would be of interest to note that this was the year in which Dr. Hornburg's medicine was confiscated and buried and the Second edition of Organon of Medicine was published.

Hartmann was reported to the Dean of the Medical Faculty Counsellor Rosenumueller, as foreign candidate for a higher degree. But the Dean died very soon and Hartmann neglected to repeat his request to the new Dean thinking that the new Dean must be knowing of his request from the papers which he had submitted previously to the Dean's office.

In the mean while he started practising although he was not entitled to do so legally.

It would be of interest to note that after Prince Schwarzenberg's death (about whom it was propagated that he had died under Hahnemann's treatment) Hahnemann was forced to leave Leipsic, and homoeopaths were the centre of attacks from all sides.

Hartmann who by then has a reputation as an advocate and admirer of homoeopathy was very soon reported against to Medical Counsellor Dr. Clarus by Dr. Kohlrush.

Hartmann then left Leipsic on New Years' day, 1821 to Berlin to continue further studies but was very much disappointed as he was late for the session which had started in November.

So he started for his home town Delitsch where his father died six days after his arrival and mother six weeks later.

Hartmann, at least, got his colloquium in 1821 after a successful examination from Dresden under the Royal Councillors Dr. Leowordi and Dr. Kreysig.

HOMOEOPATHIC PRACTICE

Hartmann settled in Zschopau as a practising physician. In 1826 he moved to Leipsic and started his homoeopathic practice there. Very soon he became very popular and the most sought after physician of Leipsic for his cures.

CONTRIBUTIONS

Hartmann was a homoeopath to the core of his heart and a faithful follower of Hahnemann but he "preserved certain unprejudiced soberness which casued him to continue aslo his other studies." Probably this was the reason, he nerve faltered in criticising Hahnemann on many matters where he thought it justified.

He played a chief role in the establishment of **Leipsic Homoeopathic Hosptial** and also worked there as chief physician.

Franz Hartmannn was on of the founders of Allgemeins Homoeopathische Zeitung, a weekly Gazette of homoeopathy. He continued to edit it till his last days. He contributed a series of articles on different drugs of our Materia Medica.

DIED

His constitution was naturally feeble and had hydrotheorax for many years. He died at 9 a.m on 10th October, 1853.

He was survived by his widow and four children. His eldest son was a homoepath and practiced in Norwich.

WRITINGS

1828 : Practical Experience in the Domain of Homoeopathy. Part-I, The Use of Nux Vomica in Disease, according to Homoeopathic Principles.

1830 : *Dietetis for Everybody* presented according to Homoeopathic Principles.

1830 : *Dietetics for the Sick* who subject themsleves to Homoeopathic Treatmnet.

1831-32 : *Therapy of Acute Diseases,* elaborated according to Homoeopathic Principles. Two Vols.

1832-53 : Co-editor of *Allgemeine homoeopathische Zeitung.* Editor of Caspari's Domestic Physician, Homoeo-

		pathic Pharmacopolea. Pocket Companion for Newly Married.
1833-34	:	Co-editor, *Year Book of the Homoeopathic Hospital at Leipsic.*
1835	:	Part-II. The Use of the Medicines, Aconitum napellus. Bryonia alba and Mercurius according to Homoeopathic Principles.
1839	:	Co-editor, *Journal fur hom. Arzneimittellehre.*
1846-55	:	*Special Therapy of Acute and Chronic Diseases according to Homoeopathic Principles.*
1850	:	My experiences and observations about homoeopathy, in 8th issues of Allg. Hom. Zeit.
1852	:	*Diseases of Children and their Treatment, according to the Homoeopathic System.*

SOURCE MATERIALS

1. **Richard Haehl :** *Samuel Hahnemann, Life and Work.* Vol. - I & II.
2. **T. L. Branford :** *The Pioneer Practititoners of Homoeopathy.*
3. *Life and Letters of Hahnemann.*
4. *North American Journal of Homoeopathy,* 1853 : P. 560, 1854 : P. 184.
5. *Philadelphia Journal of Homoeopathy,* Vol. II, P. 640.
6. *The British Journal of Homoeopathy,* 1854 : P. 150, 1874 : P. 453, 455.
7. *North Western Journal of Homoeopathy.* Vol. IV, P. 158.
8. *Medical Counsellor,* 1886 : P. 196, 238.
9. **Mahendra Singh :** *Samuel Hahnemann, A Biographical Monument and Chronology.*

Dr. J.N. Hazra

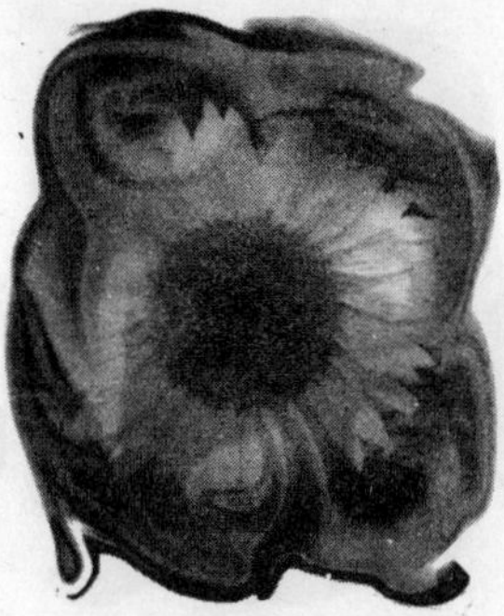

Whenever a homoeopath will think about Agra, the name of late Dr. Hażra will linger on his mind. A true Hahnemannian in approach. The efficacy and effectiveness of his treatment carried the banner of Homoeopathy to distant places of U.P. and nearby states.

Dr. Charles Julius Hempel

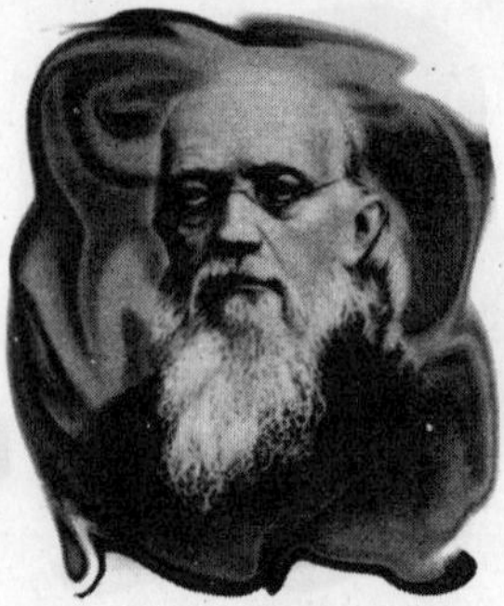

Born : 05-09-1811 **Died : 24-09-1879**

Homoeopathic history is full of dedicated men who spearheaded the new healing art to different lands of different people; of men who at the cost of great personal sacrifice devoted themselves to its practice; of men who enriched it by incorporating new drugs, new principles of remedy-selection and new pharmaceutical methods; of men who were able to bring new converts to its fold; of men who were great teachers and academicians. We are indebted to each and all of them, and they shall be remembered with gratitude by generations after generations of the students, teachers and practitioners of the human medicine, Homoeopathy. But few of us are conscious and fewer still realise the importance and the role of those very few who by their translations of the textbooks and other writings from German to English or in any other language brought homoeopathy to the heads and homes where these writings would have never entered had they remain locked up on the language of original writing. Few names shine with brilliance in this area of homoeopathic activities and brightest of them all is that of Dr. Charles Julius Hempel, the king amongst translators of our literary heritage from the language of the pathfinder to the language of the faithful followers.

BIRTH

Charles Julius Hempel was born on 5th of September in 1811 at Solingen, a manufacturing town, famous for small tools including the internationally famous solingen-knives. Solingen is very near to Cologne which was in Prussia.

EDUCATION

He received collegiate education in his country inspite of the poverty and economic hardship of his family but only because of the determination and sacrifices of his parents and his own dedication and diligence.

At the age of 21 years he went to Paris and was attracted to the charms and fame of the internationally famous teachers like Theward, Gay-Lussac, Michelet and others. He received a paltry help from his parents and executed his studies by his own earnings.

His pleasant manners and diligence soon attracted the attention of one of his teachers Mr. Michelet, who was busy in compiling the history of France. Hempel was soon accepted as a member of the Michelet family and while the pupil assisted the teacher in his literary works, the teacher in turn remained always helpful and kind to the young pupil and after completion of his studies secured a profitable employment for him as a tutor.

In 1835, at the young age of 24 years, he immigrated to United States of America and settled in New York. His intelligence, hard working nature and pleasant disposition stood him well again in need and he was accepted as a friend and house guest for 2 years of a well-to-do Italian emigrant Maroncelli, and received love and care of other Italian refugees. He learned English and Italian and soon acquired distinct proficiency in these languages. His views on political and social matters also took a definite shape at this stage. His knowledge of languages procured for him many employments and brought him in close contact with many young writers, journalists and other literary men, many of whom acquired great fame in course of time.

After about 7 years stay in New York he matriculated from the Medical Department of the University of New York and in 1845, at the age of 34 years, on 1st of March, graduated from the same university. His thesis for graduation was "ECLECTICISM IN MEDICINE OR A CRITICAL REVIEW OF THE TEACHING OF MEDICAL DOCTRINES". It was a comparison of different schools of medicine and a frank admission of his faith and preference of homoeopathy.

The glimpses of the kindness of providence on destiny and course of homoeopathy are few. The unseen hands of providence were guiding this matured, hardworking German young man towards homoeopathy, where many tasks were urgently waiting for a person of his sincerity, proficiency in German, English, French and Italian languages and most of all, a maturity in wisdom.

The literature of homoeopathy in 1845 was neither much developed nor available to all the readers of English language.

Till 1825 English language, especially in U.S.A., had only one publication, viz., CHARACTERISTICS OF HOMOEOPATHY and that too in a very poor English. Dr. Constantine Hering landed on American soil in 1833 and a devoted and capable group consisting of Dr. Gray, Hull and others was soon formed which proved to be highly significant for the homoeopathic literature in English language and for the spread of homoeopathy in the U.S.A., Great Britain and other English speaking areas of globe. Within 12 years 43 books, lectures and pamphlets were published. The famous of which were Hering's DOMESTIC PHYSICIAN (1835), Hahnemann's ORGANON OF MEDICINE (1836), Jahr's MANUAL OF HOMOEOPATHIC MEDICINE (1836), Jahr's HOMOEO PHARMACOPOEIA AND POSOLOGY (1842), of these Organon and Jahr's New Manual were annotated reprints of British translations.

In short homoeopathic literature was more or less confined to German language and the light of homoeopathy was very gradual in reaching the English speaking lands. The new world, America needed English literature on homoeopathy.

Hempel with his knowledge of languages and heroic devotion was perfectly fit for the job.

He did a difficult, honest and competent job and many of the widely acclaimed books of Hahnemann and other German stalwarts were translated and published in English.

MARRIAGE

In 1855, Dr. Hempel was married to Mrs. Mary E. Calder of Grand Rapids, Michigan and in 1856 he accepted the Chair of Materia Medica in The Homoeopathic Medical College of Philadelphia and shifted to Philadelphia. He resigned his post by the end of 1859 and returned to Grand Rapids where he spent the rest of his life with the exception of occasionally visiting the East and a year (1870-1871) spent in Europe.

Although Dr. Hempel had a considerably large practice, he continued his literary works with undiminishing zeal and at the cost of much personal loss.

In early part of 1879 his foot slipped while getting into a carriage and he fell backward and received a trauma on sacrum by the edge of the board on side-walk. There was no pain at that time but within a few months he was afflicted with an attack of paralysis of lower extremities. He never recovered completely from his paralysis. Fate struck him another serious blow. His vision started to fail him. He was accustomed to work in late hours of night using bright gas light. He used to allot himself a task of certain pages for translation everyday and he never took rest till the day's allotted task was accomplished.

When his eyes began to trouble him he increased the time and amount of his literary works. He could not be convinced of the hopelessness of the condition of his eyes even after hearing the opinions of the best opticians of U.S.A. and Europe. He was determined to finish as much work as could be done before he became completely bedridden and invalid. He was a very dedicated and determined man. He returned from Europe in 1871 but his health was seriously impaired. He was breaking down slowly but constantly. Upto 1874 he could walk in the city with the assistance of a strong cane, his devoted nurse and friend but soon his walks were restricted to the veranda of his home and ultimately he was completely bedridden and about the same time he became totally blind.

While his body was forced to bed and the outside world was shut from his vision his active brain and strong will refused to surrender. Completely paralyzed, suffering from serious pain and shut off from the outside world, he started dictating his books and in 1876 the second edition of his "Science of Homoeopathy" was published.

His only desire was to prepare an enlarged 3rd edition of his Materia Media. He was convinced that his manner of teaching Materia Medica was best and he wanted to give a clear understanding of the subject and his interest at this stage of his life centered around this work. He was so feeble that his head needed support from others, pain racked in every inch of his frail body, wasted to the very skeleton, he accomplished his desire. On 16th of September, 1879, the preface of this work was read to him. He made some corrections and he asked that the words "All Ready For The Printer" be written over it.

At that time he was suffering from severe cold and he alone realised that the end was indeed very close and waiting.

We believe that death is less painful to those who are testing chilly waters of the dark rivers than it is to the heart-broken friend, who witnesses the intensity of the struggle, and realise that we can do nothing but smooth the pillow of the dying one and pray that the end to such comrades-in-arms come soon because in their death they become graceful, milestones and lighthouse of history.

He, who had labored hard throughout his life, and lastly without sight and with a palsied, weary body was perhaps glad to be free from the shackles of an invalid body which had chained him to the invalid's couch, when in the midnight of September 24th, 1879 the final scene of the drama of an eventful and heroic life, worldly life drew to a close. He was probably ready and waiting for summons from the realm of unknown, very secure in his knowledge that his works, and his translations were to remain as his monument with an epitaph written from his unwavering determination and hardwork.

ANALYSIS & EVALUATION OF THE MAN & HIS WORKS

Samuel Lilienthal, the grand master of homoeopathic therapeutics, wrote "It is generally admitted that Hempel is the father of the homoeopathic literature of this country and that, as such, his labors have been of unestimable value to the school. Yet, few men have been more frequently misunderstood, more bitterly criticised and more persistently misrepresented".

Hempel was subjected to vigorous attacks and criticism on two counts. The first related to his translations.

Hempel's translation of Hahnemann's Materia Medica Pura of 1632 pages in 1846, was a sincere and Himalayan effort. But after few years Dr. Richard Hughes of Britain pointed out some of the inaccuracies in his translations and to common homoeopaths, ignorant of the delicacies and difficulties of translations, it struck as awful. Since then uncharitable remarks were often made about Hempel.

We feel that Hempel's criticism was more pungent than necessary and there appears to be involvement of a some personal idiosyncrasies. His standing as a translator was established beyond all doubts after his translation of the literary works of the German laureate Schiller.

We have also to understand that the task of a translator is frequently an exceedingly difficult one; the extent of the difficulty is better appreciated by them who know some languages and have attempted to translate from one language to the other. It is also a fact that no language presents more difficulties in translating than the German, and Hahnemann's style of writing is not only complicated prose of very very long sentences but he uses same words to denote different senses in many places. Dr. F.W. Hunt said, "The task then of rendering into good English the long and exceedingly complicated sentences of Hahnemann is simply appalling a vervatim translation would result in an English text, nearly as unintelligible as the original German; and a free translation is always, in the very nature of things, open to criticism." Dudgeon, who has been acclaimed as the best translator of Hahnemann's works, wrote in the translator's Preface of Organon of Medicine, "I am indebted to Dr. Richard Hughes for several emendations of my first translation, whereby the author's meaning has been rendered more exact and clearer." This proves that his first edition was not as 'exact' or as 'clearer'. But about this translation of Dudgeon Dr. Conrad Wesselhoeft, another English translator of Organon of Medicine, wrote in the preface of his translation of Organon of Medicine "Although the American edition have served their purpose, a careful comparison with the original work soon leads to the conviction that justice was not always done to it. The translation, though free in paraphrase, often obscures the sense by unsuccessful rendering of the quaintness of the author's style, and of his involved sentences. " He cities many examples of inaccuracies to prove his point.

The second reason for Hempel's criticism was his outspoken views on many matters and his attempt to introduce an element of scientific attitude into homoeopathic principles and literature. His teaching embodied the following points:

"The law of homoeopathy is a natural law and is universal; the applications of this law in the selection of a remedy constitutes the homoeopathic physician.

The medicinal value of a drug depends upon the presence of an inherent force, which can be recognized by its effects upon the healthy organism. This force may be made more available by splitting of the drug-molecule; but this process of splitting the drug-molecule is confined to certain limits.

The lower and medium attenuations yield the most satisfactory results in common practice. The use of high attenuations is often followed by the most gratifying success. Reports of cures made with the infinitesimals of Jenichen, Fincke, Swan and others are to be received very, cautiously.

The attenuation of remedies may be good homoeopathic practice.

The external use of drugs may be demanded in certain cases, the drug so used should always be strictly homoeopathic to the case; if so, its use will not be followed by injurious results.

Palliative treatment may become a duty of the homoeopathic physician.

Isopathy is a perversion of the purposes of God and should be discountenanced.

An acquaintance with physiology and pathology is a necessity in the study of the homoeopathic Materia Medica.

Provings of remedies should be made with appreciable doses of crude drugs; the lower attenuations may yield reliable symptoms in exceptional cases the higher the attenuation used in proving a remedy, the more cautiously must its results be accepted.

Hahnemman did not create the law of homoeopathy, he only discovered it; his authority is great, not final.

Most of these views imperfectly stated as they are, were taught by him to the last; he admitted, however, with the utmost readiness, that the single remedy should be the aim of the physician and he consented to an erasure from the forthcoming edition of the Materia Medica of every allusion, favoring the alternation of remedies.

In evaluating and suspecting the worth of the writings and views of a physician of upto the middle of the nineteenth century we have to keep in mind that many of the principles and conceptions were in their formative stages and the principles in regard to the use of high potency; alternation of remedies and external applications were being debated hotly by the faithful followers of Hahnemann. Such being the state of homoeopathy many of the ideas were not at all against the generally accepted and practiced norms of homoeopathy and many of the later stalwarts professed and preached much more damaging and nonhomoeopathic methods, yet Hempel was singled out by ultra Hahnemannians especially and the British-influenced homoeopaths for violent and unethical attacks. Lilienthal must have foreseen the future when he wrote.

"The hostility was carried to such an extent that the future student of the history of our school will be sorely puzzled to reconcile the charges made against Hempel."

Yes, it has been a very hard and strenuous work to salvage the true image of Hempel out of the rubbish and waste of scathing attacks, uncharitable remarks and exaggerated hostility towards Hempel, a dedicated worker and soldier of homoeopathy and one of our greatest ancestors.

HIS LITERARY CONTRIBUTIONS

His Own Writings

1840 : Christinthum and Civilization, ihre Wessen and Gegenseitiges Verhaltniz. (German) New York; P. 39.

: Grammar of the German Language. (Date unknown).

: Life of Christ (in German). (Date unknown).

1845 : On Eclecticism in Medicine; or, a Critical Review of the leading Medical Doctrines: an Inaugural Thesis presented at the New York University on the first of March, 1845, New York, P. 45.

: A Treatise on the use of Arnica in Cases of Contusions, Wounds, Strains, Sprains, Lacerations of the Solids, Concussions, Paralysis, Rheumatism, Soreness of the Nipples, etc. New York; P. 16.

1846 : The Homoeopathic Domestic Physician, New York; P. 184.

1851 : Reply to the Article on My Homoeopathic Domestic Physician, contained in No. 36 of the British Journal of Homoeopathy. P. 12. (Supplement to the North American Journal of Homoeopathy, Volume 1, May, 1851)

: Reply to a Critical Review of Hampel's Repertory, contained in Volume 1, No. 9, of the Philadelphia Journal of Homoeopathy. N.P.N.D. New York, 1852. P. 10. (Philadelphia Journal of Homoeopathy Volume 1, P. 467).

1853 : Complete Repertory of the Homoeopathic Materia Medica, New York; Volume 8, P. 224.

(This really constitutes the third volume, and Repertory to Jahr's Symptomen Codex, which Dr. Hempel translated from German into English in 1848).

: The Homoeopathic Domestic Physician. German Edition, New York; P. 133.

1854 : Nouvelle Homoeopathic Domestique, avec une Explication Introductofre du principle Homoeopathique, etc. New York; P. 151.

: Organon of Specific Homoeopathy; or, an Inductive Exposition of the Principles of the Homoeopathic Healing Art; Philadelphia; P. 216.

1857 : An Introductory Address delivered in the Homoeopathic Medical College of Pennsylvania, October 20, 1857. Philadelphia; P. 23.

1858 : Manual of Homoeopathic Theory and Practice; with an Elementary Treatise on the Homoepathic Treatment of Surgical Diseases. New York Second edition in 1863, reprint in 1872.

1859 : A New and Comprehensive System of Materia Medica and Therapeutics; arranged upon a Physiologico-Pathological Basis, for the use of Practitioners and Students of Medicine, New York; P. 1202. (This was reprinted in London, England).

: Hempel and Beakley's Manual of Homoeopathic Practice and Surgery.

: Hempel's Materia Medica, First Edition.

1865 : A New and Comprehensive System of Materia Medica and Therapeutics, Second Edition; P. 836.

1866 : What might and should be the Social and Political Relations of Homoeopathy to the Dominant School of Medicine. Address before the Michigan Homoeopathic Institute, June 19, P. 13.

1867 : A Lecture on Homoeopathy; Delivered before the Legislature of Michigan, Detroit: American Observer Print; P. 40. (Delivered at Lansing at the time a bill for introducing homoeopathy into Ann Arbor University was before the Legislature; Printed in American Homoeopathic Observer, Volume 4, P. 185).

1868 : The New Remedies; their Description. Pathogenetic Effects, and their Therapeutical Application in Homoeopathic Practice, New York, P. 72.

1869 : A Letter to Professor A. B. Palmer, A. M., M. D., of the University of Michigan; being a Reply to his four Lectures on Homoeopathy. Detroit, Michigan : Office of the American Homoeopathic Observer. P. 74.

1874 : The Science of Homoeopathy; or, a Critical and Synthetical Exposition of the Doctrines of the Homoeopathic School, New York; Boericke and Tafel. P. 177.

1876 : The same. 2nd Edition. Revised and enlarged, P. 200.

1880 : Materia Medica and Therapeutics arranged upon a Physiological and Pathological Basis, 3rd edition, two Volumes, Chicago: P. 796 & 912. (The Manuscript of this work was ready for the printer at the time of Dr. Hempel's death, on 24th September, 1879. Dr. Arndt edited the book, rewrote and condensed the second volume, and put the work through the press. The second volume was published in 1881).

1860 : Homoeopathy, a Principle in Nature. Its Scientific Universality Unfolded; its Development and Philosophy Explained; and its Applicability to the Treatment of Diseases Shown, Philadelphia, P. 248.

Translations

1845 : Boenninghausen on "Intermittent Fever", P. 56.

1845-46 : Hahnemann's Chronic Diseases, with clinical suggestions by Noak and Trinks. P. 1632.

1846 : Hahnemann's Materia Medica Pura, with Clinical suggestions by Noak Trinks, P. 877.

: Stapf's Additions to the Materia Medica Pura, P. 292.

: Rueckert's Therapeutics of Homoeopathy, P. 496.

1847 : Hartmann's Theory of Acute Diseases, etc., P. 476.

: Raue's Organon of the Specific Healing Art. P. 220.

: Boenninghausen's Therapeutic Pocket book for Homoeopathic Physicians, P. 504.

1848 : Jahr's New Manual (Symptomen-Codex), P. 2003.

1849 : Hartmann's Theory of Chronic Diseases, 12mo., P. 258.

1850 : Jahr's New Homoeopathic Pharmacopoeia and Posology, P. 359.

: Jahr's Repertory of the Skin Symptoms, P. 515.

: Jahr's Clinical Guide, P. 408.

: The same; 2nd edition. Revised and considerably enlarged, P. 216.

1854 : Teste's Materia Medica, translated from the French.

1856 : Tessier on Pneumonia.

: Tessier on Asiatic Chlora.

1857 : Jahr's Diseases of Females and Infants at the Breast, translated from the French.

1862 : Lutze's Manual of Homoeopathic Thera-peutics.

1868 : Jahr's Venereal Diseases.

: Jahr's Forty Years' Practice.

1869 : Jahr's Clinical Guide.

: Baehr's Science of Therapeutics.

Year Not Ascertained

: Mure's Brazilian Provings.
Jahr's Diseases of the Mind.

: Raue's Organon.
Hartmann's Diseases of Children.

: Rueckert's Therapeutics.
Schacfer's Homoeopathic Veterinary.
Schiller's Works (on German literature).

: Jahr's Skin Diseases.

: Jahr's Nervous Diseases.

: Gollman's Diseases of the Sexual Organs.

Many of these works are more than mere translations. Baehr's work for instance, contains very copious editions from Kafka.

Dr. Constantine Hering

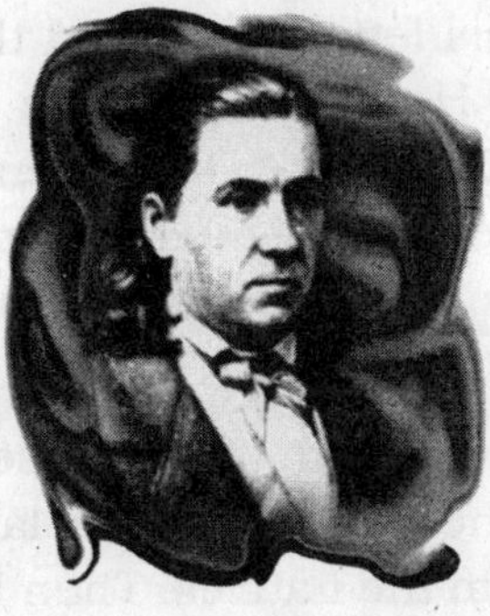

Born : 01-01-1800 **Died : 23-07-1880**

The history of homoeopathy is made of many people, but Constantine Hering stands as a Colossus. "He was a man of iron constitution, who never seemed to tire or to need time for rest and relaxation". He was a worthy successor to Hahnemann.

Hering, M.D., was born on the 1st of January, 1800, at Oschatz, Saxony. From an early age he had an extreme desire to investigate all things. At the age or nine or ten he had found the Caterpillar Sphynx Atropos on his father's grapevine, which was the beginning of his studies in natural history. Under the guardianship of the eminent Surgeon, Robbi, he entered the University of Leipzig. In 1826, he graduated with his medical degree from the university of Wurzburg.

He received a dissecting wound in his right index finger, in 1821. Doctors advised amputation of his finger, but he refused to do so. One of his friend persuaded him to try a ridiculously minute dose of *Arsenicum*. The symptoms of recovery appeared and Hering was cured of his ailment. Homoeopathy saved his finger. Hering said "the last obstacles placed between my eyes and the rising sun of the new healers are vanished. The finger is still my own." Hering wrote his first letter to Hahnemann in 1824, and Hahnemann replied, "your active zeal for the beneficial art delights me.... I would like to become better acquainted with you."

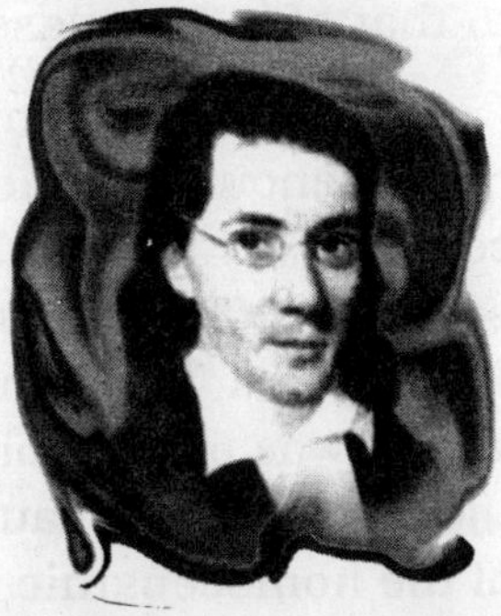

Hering worked as an instructor in natural history for a very brief period. Then he received a commission from the king of Saxony to serve as the botanist on a botanical and zoological expedition to Surinam. Hering

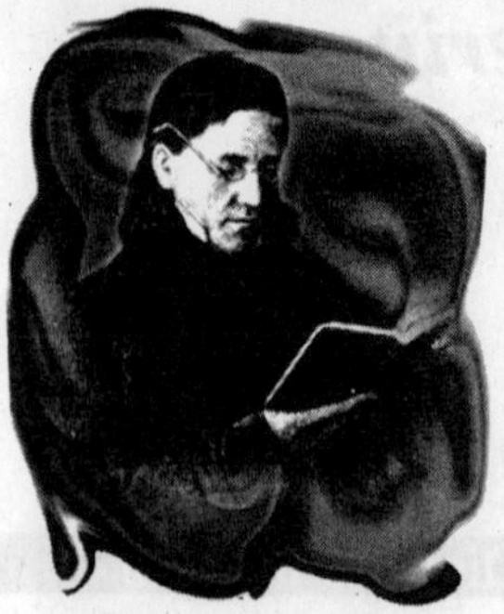

sent his first letter to staff's *Archive,* in 1827; when the court physician came to know about this letter, he asked the king to send a letter to Hering, telling him to tend to his botanical duties and to let medical matters alone. Hering resigned his appointment and settled, as a homoeopathic physician, in Surinam.

In 1828, in Surinam, Hering became interested in the use of snake poisons as remedies. He milked the venom from a large surukuku or bush master which he got from the natives. Then he triturated the venom with sugar of milk to obtain a homoeopathic potency.

A translation of Hering's own account of his first meeting with the famed bush master snake was published in *Simillimum,* in 1991. According to Hering, he was living in Paramaribo, Surinam, and had been looking for a good snake specimen. The natives brought him one that had been run over by a cart at the edge of town. Hering untied the snake and noticed that it was alive. He extracted some venom and began to triturate it with sugar of milk. Accidentally he ingested some, and the first proving began. He had done 104 provings upon himself. He introduced the remedies — *Lachesis, Psorinum* and *Glonoine.*

Hering met a young German - American missionary, George Bute, in Paramaribo. Bute learned homoeopathy from Hering and returned to the United States to practice in Pennsylvania. Hering joined his practice in Philadelphia, in 1833. Few months after his arrival in Philadelphia, he was approached by Wesselhoeft, Detwiller, and Romig, who were representing the Homoeopathic Society of Northampton and Counties Adjacent, with a proposal to establish a homoeopathic school. They requested Hering to join the school as the President and Principal Instructor at a salary equal to that of a first class Allentown Clergyman.

A stock company was formed, and a number of Subscribers raised enough money to buy a tract of land in Allentown. The cornerstone was laid, on 27th of May, for the first homoeopathic school — The North American Academy of the Homoeopathic Healing Art. This school is also known as Allentwon Academy. The school was opened on Hahnemann's birthday — April 10, 1835. All the courses were taught in German language. It was the language of the homoeopathic literature at that time.

The school lasted only for six years; it was ceased when Wesselhoeft moved to Boston in 1842. The school published both Hahnemann's *Organon* and Jahr's *Manual* in the English language. The school was ceased due to the financial crash, the banker with whom the school's endowment fund was deposited made a bad failure, and the money was lost.

In 1831 Hering was married to Charlotte Van Kemper, in Surinam. A son was born to them whom they named John. His wife died in 1831.

Hering married again to Marianne Husmann, in 1834, in America. Four children were born to Marianne and Hering. His second wife, Marianne, died in 1840. Hering returned to Germany in 1845, there he met Therese Bucheim, he married her and returned to the United States in 1846. From this marriage there were eight children, six of whom survived him.

According to Knerr, Hering's household was always full of life. There were conversations constantly after dinners, either around the table or in the garden, under the grape arbor.

Knerr describes a meeting of Hering and Dunham where Dunham asked the questions and Hering gave the answers, while Lilienthal (and Knerr) sat and listened.

Dr. George Norton recalled Hering's chief pleasure and relaxations from work were the "meetings on Sunday afternoon, when a circle of old friends assembled in his reception room, and over cigars and coffee compared experiences and discussed various subjects. Neither hot, cold, nor stormy weather interfered with these social gatherings."

Hering's favourite saying was, "change of occupation is rest."

Homoeopathic pharmacy was the another area of Hering's interest and which he maintained until his death. It was Hering who convinced Dr. Samuel Dubs to make the first "decimal potencies" in the United States. Hering also trained Rudolph Tafel as his personal pharmacist.

On July 23, 1880, Hering saw a patient at 6 o'clock and had supper with his family, talked for an hour, and then retired to his study to work on volume four of the *'Guiding Symptoms'*. He rang up his wife, a little before 10 o'clock, and said he was having difficulty in breathing. His wife sent for the doctor. By the time Dr. Rane arrived, he could do nothing but turn and walk away in grief.

The funeral was held on July 28, 1880, the 52nd anniversary of his first *Lachesis* proving.

Dr. Lilienthal said, at a memorial service, "Dr. Hering died in harness. At six o'clock on the evening of his death he made his last prescription".

Hering was a voracious writer. In Bradford's Bibliography we find 352 items under his name including his five best known books:

1835 Domestic physician.

1867 Comparative Materia Medica.

1873 Materia Media.

1875 Analytical Therapeutics.

1877 Condensed Materia Medica.

1880 The Guiding Symptoms of Materia Medica. This book was published in 10 volumes. Hering was working on the third Volume of his Guiding Symptoms of the Materia Medica when he died.

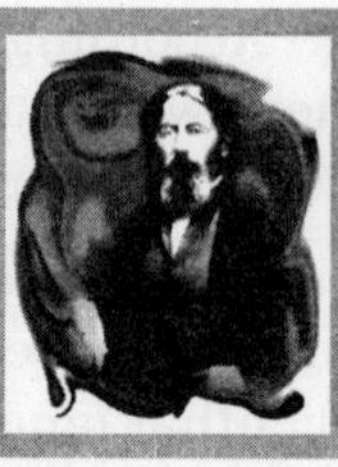

He was editor of the *North American Homoeopathic Journal,* from 1851 to 1853; the *Homoeopathic News,* from 1854 to 1856; the *American Homoeopathic Materia Medica* from 1867 to 1871.

Dr. Hering is also famous for the *Law of Direction of Cure,* which is as follows: Cure takes place from above downward; from within outward; from a more important organ to a less important organ. Symptoms disappear in the reverse order of their appearance, the first to appear being the last to go.

Dr. John Martin Honigberger

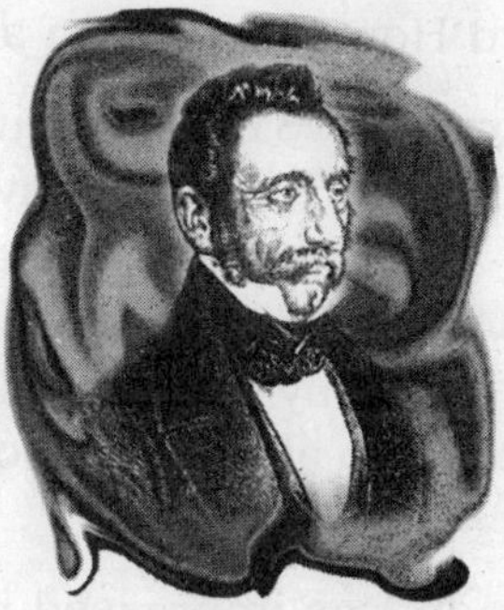

Every serious Indian Homoeopath might know the name of Dr. John Martin Honigberger who received, possibly the first ever, official patronage to practice Homoeopathy in South East Asia in the Durbar of Maharaja Ranjit Singh of erstwhile-undivided Punjab. There are varying versions about his Nationality. Some suggest he was German, few suggest French, yet others say Hungarian, still another group say Romanian. Some authors quote his native place as *Pennsylvania*, Romania. The country of origin of Honigberger has been mentioned differently at different places in the references on the origin of Homoeopathy in India including the Websites.

With a view to correct position, an effort was made to get the factual position.

Few sketches of Dr. Martin Honigberger are exhibited at the Maharaja Ranjit Singh Museum at Amritsar, Punjab. The following note is written under one such exhibit.

"Honigberger was born at Kronstadt (Transylvania), Hungary around the year 1795. He travelled widely before coming to Punjab in 1829. Introduced to Maharaja Ranjit Singh by General Allard. He was appointed as Physician at his Court and given the charge of the gun powder and ammunition factory besides providing the Maharaja with one of the strongest potions ever made in the world."

"Honigberger was very close to the French Officers and like them took interest in history and archaeology. While on his way back to Europe in 1833, he made extensive excavations at Hadda (near Jalalabad) and Kabul bringing an impressive collection of coins and artefacts back to Vienna, Paris and London. He returned to Lahore in 1838 and attended to Prince Nau Singh after his fatal accident on 5th March 1840."

Please note that there is no mention about his successful treatment of the Maharaja with Dulcamara for his vocal cord paralysis nor of the word Homoeopathy in any of these exhibits.

He left his native town in 1815. He visited Jerusalem and as a Physician to the Governor of Tocat he travelled with him to Asia Minor. His first patient at Lahore was the adopted son of General Allard. His fame spread only when he treated and cured some soliders who had been bitten by a mad jackal and were beginning to show signs of hydrophobia, after some soldiers had already died of the bite.

Maharaja Ranjit Singh was impressed by him when he treated his favourite horse of its bad ulcers of the leg. The Maharaja had come to have great confidence in him and made him accept the management of a gunpowder manufactory and also a gunstock establishment. Being homesick, Honigberger went back in 1834. Next year he went to Paris and met Dr. Hahnemann. He bought a large quantity of homoeopathic medicines from Hahnemann's Pharmacist, Lehmann of Kothen.

In the year 1836, he happened to go to Vienna and caught an infection of choldera which was raging there. He saved himself by taking Ipecac, every half an hour. He was impressed greatly by the results of homoeopathic medicine both on himself and others.

He decided to start his practice at Constatinople. He treated cases of plague with Ignatia. He was led to use it because he saw Armenians there wearing a string tied to a bean of *Ignatia* and it seemed to give them protection where so many people were dying every day.

He also treated a case of haemorrhage with *Aranea-diadema* which brought him both name and fame. It is said that he had a very lucrative practice.

On Learning that Maharaja Ranjit Singh wanted him back, he reached Lahore in 1839 in the company of General Venture after an adventurous journey.

After the death of the Maharaja his position and influence wanted till Sardar Jawahar singh came to power, and restored him to his former position as Court Physician and Director of the gun-powder mill. In 1849, the Punjab was annexed by Sir Henry Lawrence. With the abolition of the 'Singh Darbar' he had to relinquish his post. He was granted a pension. Later he returned to his country.

It is not known when he died, but his life was full of adventure and pioneering. He was the first man to introduce the name Dr. Samuel Hahnemann and his healing art to India.

There is also no mention about being witness to the murder of the Maharaja in the book — *"Thirty Five Years in the East"*, by Dr. Honigberger, first published in 1852 from London. In this book, he says of being present when the Maharaja gave up his temporal life. The book describes in detail of witnessing the brutal murder of the son of Maharaja and the organized onslaught of the Great Kingdom by the evil forces. (Can the historians look into whether the Maharaja was killed or had passed away and whether omitting the contribution of Honigberger to Indian Homoeopathy was deliberate).

Though out of context, let us look into the writings of Honigberger himself about the first officially recorded Homoeopathic treatment in India. This gives a glimpse of the beginning of Homoeopathy in the South East Asia.

"Arriving at Lahore, I found my former patron, the Maharaja Ranjit Singh, seated on a chair, with swollen feet, and making himself understood by gestures and sing with his hands, his organ of speech being paralysed to such a degree that the was not able to utter a single articulate sound."

Form time to time I had occasion to relate many of he cures effected by the new method of Homoeopathy by aid which I had cured myself in Vienna of the cholera, and lately in Hindustan of the Plague."

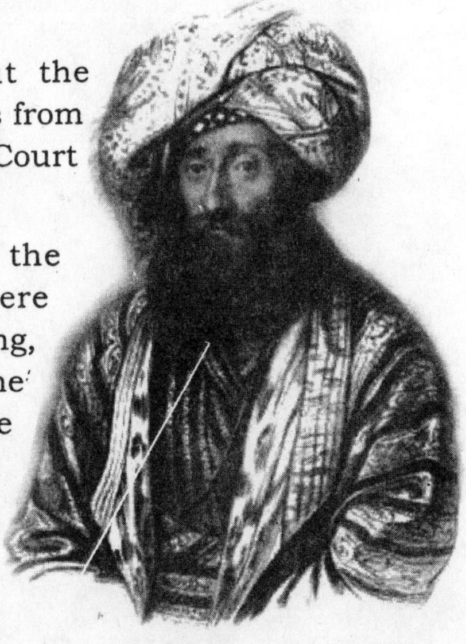

He describes in detail about the preparation of Dulcamara potencies from the mother tincture in front of the Court Physicians in subsequent paras.

"During the preparation of the medicine, some persons who were standing by could not forbear smiling, and the Faquir himself was of the opinion that such a minute dose could not be hurtful, should it even by supposed to be poison. But what was the result? ON the first day, there was no visible amelioration in the health of the Maharaja, on the second day he felt somewhat better, and on the third day, he was in such a merry humour that at five o'clock in the afternoon, he ordered the minister Dhyan Singh, to put a pair of gold bracelets on my arms, valued at five hundred rupees, in his own presence and in that of the durbar."

The sad part of this history is, inspite of such remarkable achievement, which paved the foundation for official recognition of Homoeopathy as a system of medicine in India, Dr. Honigberger met the worst humiliation of his life in the same durbar itself from the practitioners of his time. (As this is not relevant to the topic, details are not attempted).

Dr. Honigberger writes about his Nationality in his book:

"Thirty five years spent in Asia - travelling from my native country (Transylvania) by way of levant, Egypt, Arabia and Persia, to India, residing in several years in the Punjab and returning by Afghanistan..........."

Transylvania is presently in Romania. Hence, the great Dr. Honigberger was a Romanian from Transylvania region. (And as he lived for several years and had a Kashmiri wife and daughters, therefore, Indianised!).

Dr. Richard Hughes

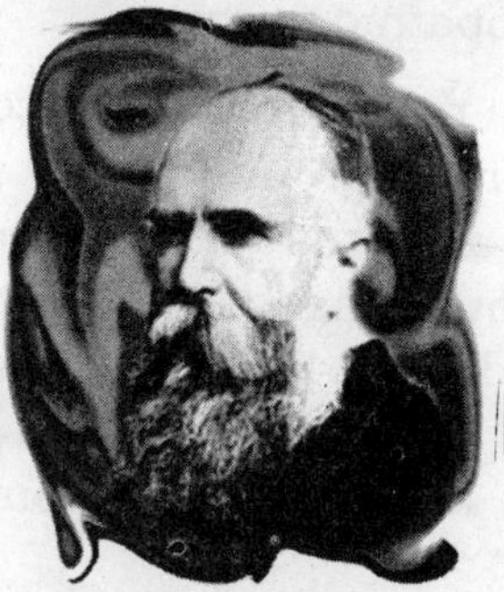

Born : 1836 **Died : 09-04-1902**

Dr. Bushrod James had said about Richard Hughes that, “His personality was extremely wining; his voice rich, clear, and steady; his eyes beautiful in youth with the merry turinkle of fun or the soft glow of sympathy as occasion required, and always pure and true. He was tall and slender in figure, and as age drew on he leaned forward slightly, not as with years, however, but as though his tender ministrations to human sufferers had drawn him down to listen. He was handsome, with no shade of vanity; genial and gleefully able to either give or take a joke, without a gleam of undue levity. He advanced his ideas with force, yet showed graceful respect to those who disagreed with his views, and his knowledge, gained by the utmost concentration and research, has been accepted as correct even by those who combated some of his theories.”

Hughes received his education at Edinburgh, Scotland, but practiced in Brighton, England. A year before his death, he moved to Albany, Guilds Ford, to become the Catholic Apostolic Church Pastor.

In 1867, he wrote, *“Manual of Pharmacodynamics”* and *“Manual of Therapeutics”*. He worked as an officer for the British Homoeopathic Society. He was the editor of the British Journal of Homoeopathy. He also edited the six volume *Cyclopedia of Drug Pathogenesy* and worked with T.F. Allen on his 10 volume *Encyclopedia.*

While compiling the *Cyclopedia,* Hughes decided to eliminate all the proving symptoms gained from the drugs taken at potencies above the 6c. He said that, “it is necessary to understand the pathology created by the remedies on the organic level and it is this pathology level which has to be treated.”

Section-H : Dr. Hughes, Richard

Thomas Skinner, a critic of Hughes' approach, said that, "His concept of low potencies was ideal for those who did not wish to stray far from their allopathic training."

J.H. Clarke said, in regard to Hughes concept of low potencies, "If it were put forward on the grounds that it meets the requirements of those who have not acquired the necessary gifts to practice the higher grades and not being a scientific improvement on the Hahnemannian method, then little be said against it." John Clarke was one of his most promising medical student. Hughes had appointed him as his assistant editor on the *British Journal of Homoeopathy,* in 1883.

In 1868, Hughes' *Pharmacodynamics* was published. About his *Pharmacodynamics,* Burnett said, "We all fed on it." Hughes' work on materia medica will always remain very valuable. Hughes died on the 9th of April, 1902.

SECTION-J .... Page 167 to 168

J-1 ***Dr. Jaisoorya, N.M.***
(Born: 26-09-1899 / Died: 1964) 168

Dr. N.M. Jaisoorya

Born : 26-09-1899

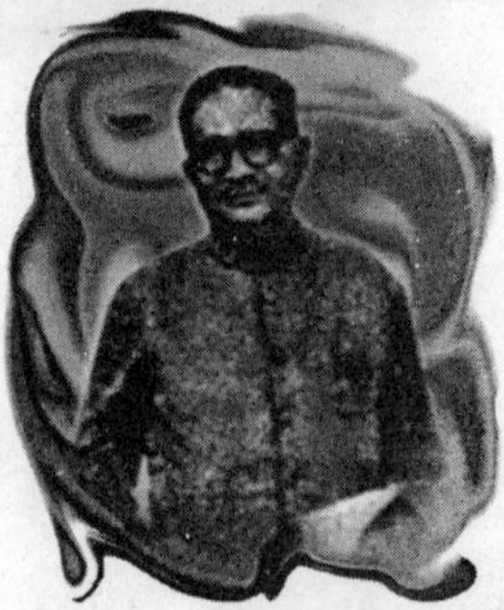

Died : 1964

Dr. N.M. Jaisoorya was born to illustrious parents, Maj. Mutyala Govindrajulu Naidu and Sarojini Naidu at Hyderabad on September 26, 1899. He fought for the recognition of the homoeopathy system of medicine in our country, especially in Andhra Pradesh. He was the founder and the first President of Andhra Pradesh Homoeopathic Association. He was elected as a president on two occasions of the All India Homoeopathic Medical Association, Delhi. He made valuable recommendations to the Government of India and to the State Governments on the teaching of homoeopathy and on the establishment of homoeopathic hospitals.

Dr. Jaisoorya opened a Leprosy Investigating and Treatment Centre in 1937 at Zahirabad, which is thriving well and catering cures for ailing individuals.

Dr. Jaisoorya was almost planning to go to Russia for the treatment of his eyes where he wanted to learn the technique of tissue therapy in the Filtoy's clinic, but death snapped him away in 1964 and deprived us all of the supreme opportunities of knowing of various allied branches of medicine.

SECTION-K .... Page 169 to 184

K-1 ***Dr. Kent, James Tyler***
(Born: 31-03-1849 / Died: 06-06-1916) 170

Dr. James Tvler Kent

Born : 31-03-1849

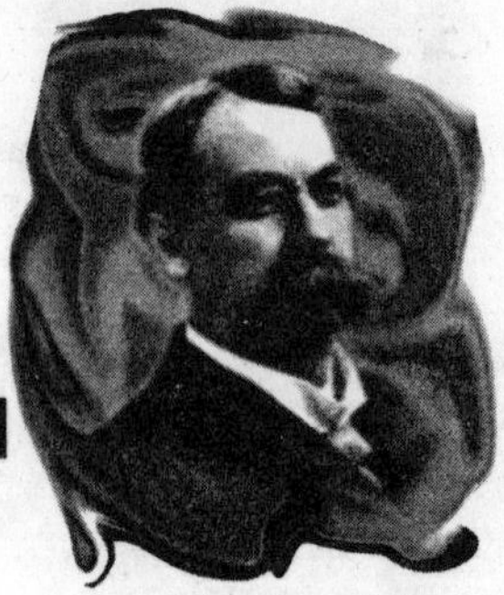

Died : 06-06-1916

BIRTH

On March 31st 1849, at Woodhull, New York State, in the United States of America, a son, James Tyler, was born to Stephen Kent and his wife Caroline.

EDUCATION

This son was to attend the Franklin School in Prattsburgh for his primary schooling, and to go on to the Woodhull Academy in the town of his birth to complete his secondary education. At the age of nineteen, James Tyler kent graduated from Madison, University at Hamilton, New York State, with a Ph.D. degree; this was followed two years later by that of A.M. from the same university. He then went on to study medicine at the Faculty of Bellevue Medical College where he passed his final examination brilliantly and qualified as a doctor of medicine. He subsequently attended two courses of lectures at the Eclectic Medical Institute at Cincinnati in the State of Ohio.

This eclectic school taught the same branches of medicine as in Europe; thatomy, histology, physiology, pathological biatomy, etc., and also offered the same clinical teaching.

The therapeutic teaching of this Eclectic Medical Institute was much more comprehensive than that of the official allopathic school. Allopathy, Homoeopathy, Naturopathy, Chiropraxy, as well as various other methods (hence the term "Eclectic") little known or quite unknown in Europe at that time, were taught. But all subjects, and especially Homoeopathy, were taught very superficially and as a result Kent was neither impressed nor convinced by this latter therapeutic method.

Section-K : Dr. Kent, James Tyler

We must remember that such Eclectic teaching, which imparted to its students a genuine tolerance of the various therapeutic methods, although of advantage to some, caused quite serious difficulties to others, since it did not extol one method and claim its superiority over the others. Thus the student was left to make his own free choice of method according to his personal inclination or based on influences to which he had been exposed or the force of circumstance.

Although an undemonstrative man Kent adored his wife and he was deeply troubled about the worsening state of her health; a state of debility, languor, anaemia and persistent insomnia had kept her bedridden for months. It was at this time that Kent underwent a period of considerable dissatisfaction with the therapeutic methods being practiced by himself and his colleagues. Neither his own eclectic practitioners nor those of the allopathic school could bring about an improvement in his wife's condition. When it became visibly worse, Mrs Kent begged him, as a last resort, to call in a certain homoeopathic doctor, well on in years, who had been recommended to her as being highly competent. Kent looked a little askance at this suggestion as he had already consulted every physician of repute in St. Louis. Being faced with a condition which was growing every day more serious he considered it ridiculous to resort to Homoeopathy (of the kind he had been taught during the courses taken at the Eclectic Medical School), about which he was by no means convinced and whose minute dose appeared to him to be absurd for a case as serious as that of his wife's. However, he bowed to her insistence, at the same time expressing a wish to be present at the consultation.

The homoeopath, Dr. Phelan, goatee-ed and dressed in a frock coat, arrived one afternoon in his barouche. He questioned the patient for over an hour, asking her about her antecedents, her past illnesses, accidents, her mental state, and her fears and her carvings. He elicited from her many details regarding her likes and dislikes about food although she had complained of no digestive troubles. He asked her minute details about her indispositions, her reaction to cold and heat and to climatic and seasonal factors. Kent found the questions so odd and seemingly inappropriate that, as he leaned on the side of the bed, he could not refrain from smiling.

Having auscultated and examined the patient, Dr. Phelan asked for a glass of water and Kent brought it. He then saw Dr.

Phelan drop a few minute globules into the glass and give Mrs Kent a spoonful of the mixture. Mrs Kent was then asked to take a small spoonful every two hours until — "the homoeopath had the effrontery to say" — she went to sleep. Since for several weeks his wife had barely closed her eyes, Kent felt that the homoeopath was either an impostor or a quack and he brusquely showed him out.

Kent then went to his study, which adjoined the sickroom, to continue work on a lecture he was preparing. Two hours later, not wanting to distress his wife, he administered a spoonful of the medicine but without the least conviction as to its efficacy. He returned to his study and then became engrossed in his work that he forgot to return to Mrs Kent two hours later to give her the third dose of the medicine. It was some four hours later that he suddenly remembered his oversight. Going to his wife's room he found her in a deep and sound sleep, something long unknown to her despite her frequent and conscientious taking of drugs. Thereafter the old homoeopath paid daily calls and gradually the condition of the patient improved until she was able to get up. Within a few weeks she had recovered her health completely.

This humble homoeopathic physician had been able to achieve that which none of the eminent physicians or professors of the allopathic and eclectic schools whom Kent had consulted had not been able to do. Dr. Phelan had restored the health of Mrs Kent gently, rapidly and permanently.

Kent was deeply impressed by what he had witnessed and his naturally frank and straightforward character compelled him to apologize to his colleague; he had to confess that the scepticism he had felt at the time of the first visit had been dispelled by the improvement in his wife's condition. After her cure his views on the practice of medicine underwent a complete change. He felt sure that the improvement which he had observed taking place in his wife from day to day could not be the result of chance or coincidence and he was obliged to ask himself whether perhaps there was not some real merit in homoeopathy. The cure of his wife moved him so deeply that he determined to make a thorough investigation into this type of therapy.

Kent's intense desire to alleviate suffering led him to concentrate all the power of his vast intellect and his indomitable will to the arduous task of acquiring a deep knowledge of homoeopathy and to this end gave himself unstintingly. Under the guidance of Dr. Phelan he studied Hahnemann's *Organon* the basic treatise of homoeopathy — and worked night and day perusing everything he could lay hands on which dealt with this paradoxical method. It is also said that for weeks at a time he would sit up for the greater part of the night, enveloped in an overcoat against the cold, to devour all available literature published in America on the subject of Homoeopathy.

In whatever he undertook he mastered each step from the beginning to the end and this proved to be the case with Homoeopathy also. He was so overwhelmed by what he discovered that he decided to resign his chair of Anatomy and to give up his membership of the Eclectic National Medical Association. This was the turning point in his medical career and from this time dates his whole-hearted conversion to Homoeopathy.

Deep sincerity and an impartiality born of absolute integrity were very marked in Kent and he devoted himself, body and soul, to this new doctrine, the deep value and truth of which he was able to perceive. In particular he realized, when comparing this with the other methods he had learned, that it was the only one to offer a Law and Principles to follow as a guide in therapeutics. All other systems appeared to him to be aleatory and inconstant. While the allopathic and eclectical schools deal with consequences, Kent recognized the primary concern of homoeopathy to be, as far as possible, that of fundamental causes. He had also observed that to take action based on consequences, even though these might be highly placed on the ladder of effects, could not bring about effective amelioration, much less a cure. He had observed that every form of therapy operating on results would bring failure and for this reason he had become dissatisfied with his practice.

Now, suddenly, the case of his wife came to point out a new direction. It was during this period that he had occasion to observe the real difference between all other therapeutic methods and that of homoeopathy when practiced according to the precise instructions of the founder. His study of homoeopathy brought him such certainty and conviction that he knew no peace until he was able himself to apply this doctrine with all the conscientiousness and strictness it demanded. So, he devoted again his full time to his patients, enlightened by all he had learned, thanks to Dr. Phelan, and in a very short time his homoeopathic practice flourished.

Through exceedingly hard work he confirmed the absolute veracity of the Law of Similars and established the need for

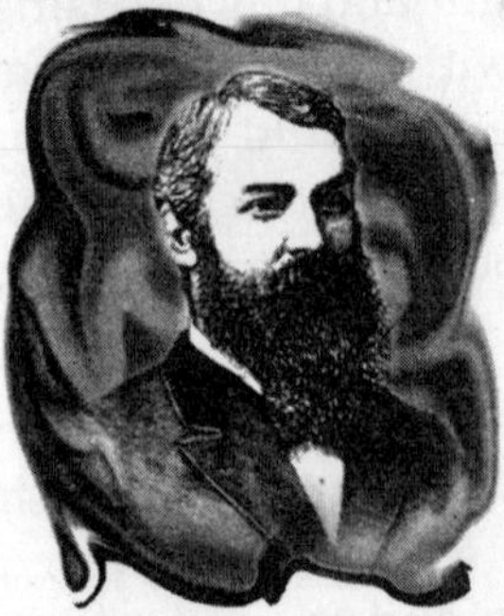

individualization. He confirmed also the unbelievable efficacy of minute doses, thanks to the process of dynamization discovered by the founder, Samuel Hahnemann.

In 1882 Kent was appointed to the Chair of Surgery at the Missouri Homoeopathic Medical College, St Louis, until the retirement in 1883 of Dr. Uhlemeyer, the Professor of Materia Medica. At that time Dr. Uhlemeyer had urged that Kent take charge of his department, since his special suitability for it was generally recognized. Kent accepted the post which he held until 1888; he left it to conduct the work of the Philadelphia Postgraduate School of Homoeopathy to which he devoted himself until the year 1899. This College had then the reputation of being the best homoeopathic school in the world. In addition to being the Dean of that institution he also taught Homoeopathic Philosophy, Repertorization and Materia Medica and he conducted an out-patient clinic. As an illustration of the activity of this clinic it may be mentioned that during the years 1896 and 1897 a total of over 34,800 consultations took place here.

While Dean of the Philadelphia Postgraduate School of Homoeopathy Kent lost his wife. In the months of sorrow which followed he plunged ever more ardently into his pioneering work about homoeopathy, performing experiments on himself and striving without respite to perfect the science and the art of this form of therapy. It was during this time that he studied and rallied to the philosophy of Swedenborg which provided him with a transcendental vision of the problem of sickness and healing. But his feet remained firmly planted on the ground and he was able to create a method which could be taught and applied for the study of symptoms and the search for the Similimum.

In 1896, some years after the death of his wife, Kent was called upon to attend a patient whom he was to treat a long time and finally marry. His second wife, Clara Louise Tobey of Philadelphia, had completed her study of medicine, first of Allopathy and then of Homoeopathy, and had become a homoeopathic practitioner. This patient had consulted the most eminent allopathic and homoeopathic physicians in the U.S.A. without benefit. All of the great homoeopathic physicians had prescribed *Lachesis,* since she had the symptoms of the remedy. Kent studied her case with the utmost care and after prolonged reflection came to the conclusion that for some years she had been engaged in a real proving of *Lachesis* which had given her, in homoeopathic terms, its medicamental miasma." If a substance whose symptoms one experiences is taken repeatedly, it may give rise to a medicamental malady which may sometimes become very serious and even incurable. Kent predicted also with complete accuracy — that the patient would exhibit lifelong symptoms of *Lachesis*. He declared she must never again touch this remedy and must henceforth take antidotes against its toxic effects.

Kent found this able and intelligent woman an inspiring helpmate and it was with her help that he was able to give the world his masterly works: *The Philosophy*, *The Materia Medica* and *The Repertory*, about which we shall speak later. The presence and sustained help of this co-worker were infinitely precious to the Master but she was unable to reduce his overwork and to restrain his indefatigable zeal in the great cause that he had undertaken, by obliging him to rest.

His renown was such that he was in demand everywhere. In 1900, on his appointment as the Dean of Dunhan Homoeopathic Medical College in Chicago, he become at the same time Professor of Homoeopathic Philosophy, Repertory and Materia Medica. At a later period he taught Materia Medica with presentation and discussion of clinical cases to the students of all the classes, from the first year to the final year, at the Hahnemann Homoeopathic Medical College, Chicago, and was appointed Dean of that college in 1905. Here he wrote to a physician on one occasion: "I am glad you are helped by my works. It is a dull time for pure homoeopathy and most of the colleges sneer at it. I am glad I have a free chance at teaching. They are all very nice to me in our Hahnemann College of Chicago. I lecture twice each week to all the four classes in the amphitheater. This gives the freshers a chance to hear my entire course as it takes four years to cover the Materia Medica. Ours is the only college in which a student is taught pure homoeopathy. It is true that much that is not true is taught by some of our teachers but I try to keep our students from absorbing the mongrelism."

Nevertheless the bitter competition at Chicago between the Hering and Dunham Medical College was painful subject among the homoeopaths and all others who were supporting those institutions. The purpose and principles of those schools were in fact the same but having two establishments with twice the personnel did nothing but double the expenses and at the same time diminish the financial support and the teaching possibilities. Negotiations were initiated between those two rival schools in 1903 and ended in a favourable agreement which permitted the incorporation of the Dunham Medical College with the Hering which was then called the Hering Medical College, of which Kent had the honour to become the President.

I must stress that the Hering College proved ultimately to be by far the best college of its kind ever established and only the purest form of homoeopathy was taught there. The student received homoeopathic instruction through all the years of his study, i.e. from the day of joining until his graduation with an M.D. degree. The student was required to study in this college for the same number of years as the allopathic student in the allopathic college. Homoeopathic philosophy, repertorization, chronic miasmata of Hahnemann and homoeopathic materia medica formed the basis of the teaching in addition to the following subjects: anatomy, physiology, histology, pathology, chemistry, toxicology, pharmacy, hygiene, dietetics, medical jurisprudence, practice of medicine, diagnosis — clinical and physical, neurology, pediatrics, dermatology, diseases of the chest, genito-urinary diseases, gynecology, obstetrics, ophthalmology, oto-rhino-laryngology, and surgery.

Three outstanding professors at the Hering Homoeopathic Medical College were Kent, H.C. Allen and J.H. Allen. The latter

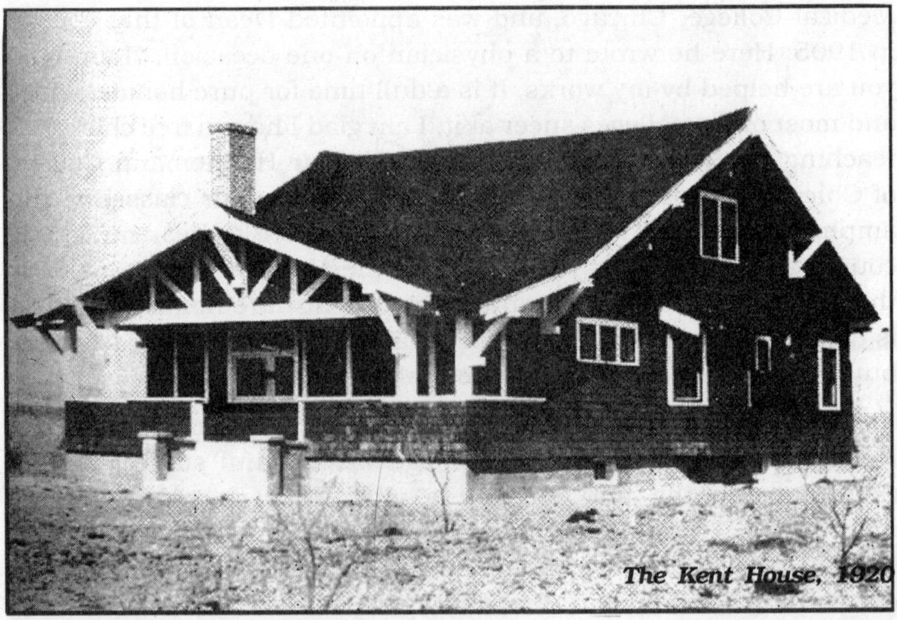

The Kent House, 1920

was Professor of "Chronic Miasmata of Hahnemann" and is the author of that most valuable work *Psora, Pseudo-Psora* and *Sycosis*. The physicians who studied at this college have done much to spread the teaching of Hahnemannian Homoeopathy. One student of Kent, Sir John Weir, lectures at the Royal London Homoeopathic Hospital in London. Another, Professor Dr. B.K. Bose, a student of the Hering Homoeopathic Medical College, still teaches in the oldest homoeopathic medical college now in existence — the Calcutta Homoeopathic Medical College and Hospital in India.

It was at this period of his life that Kent was giving the best of his knowledge in his lectures. In addition to his teaching, which took a great part of his time, he directed a polyclinic which was always very crowded, where he taught homoeopathic physicians, already well advanced in their knowledge, to detect and make a correct choice of essential symptoms in a few minutes. Because of Kent's far reaching understanding of the characteristics he was able to find the remedy at once. Kent's lectures were thronged and those in his audience who could not answer or who answered badly were not asked to do so a second time — indeed a redoubtable test for all those aspiring to become good homoeopathic physicians.

At his lectures on homoeopathic philosophy Kent would lay Hahnemann's *Organon* on the lectern and thrusting his hands under his coat tails he would expound all that his keen intellect and perspicacity had extracted when meditating upon the various sections of its 294 paragraphs. On the first section alone, the shortest of all, Kent performed over an hour's exegesis.

Hahenmann had bequeathed an Organon expressed in a condensed and rather difficult form, but Kent was able to interpret its contents and in his philosophy to present them to his students (and to the physicians of our era) in a form easy to understand. On one occasion a very scholarly and deep-thinking acquaintance had remarked to Kent, "I have read your *Philosophy* five times and I am still reading it and just now I am beginning to understand Hahnemann's *Organon*." It is he had followed in the footsteps of Hahnemann, but he had done more. He had outstripped him; he had discovered the doctrine of the Language of Revision, had shown the direction of the course of treatment immediately following the first dose and how the multiple reactions following this step should be interpreted and the patient led scientifically towards complete recovery.

Kent's exposition on "Simple Substance" is marvellous. This

"Substance" is that which is real, to distinguish it from that which is apparent. It is really the basis of all external manifestations — the permanent object of the cause of phenomena, either material of spiritual. It is not only the essence of something living extant, but it is the essence plus the existence. Although immaterial we must not consider it as non-spatial but really as an "energetic spatial".

During his lifetime Hahnemann's ideas in connection with the repetition of the dose underwent several changes; then, at the close of his life, he experimented with a new method which is described in the sixth edition of the *Organon*. This method is in fact very complicated and is not suited for practical use today, moreover, it is not able to deal with full satisfaction with the drug miasma which Hahnemann had declared, in section 76 of the sixth edition of the *Organon,* he could not tackle. "A human healing art, for the restoration to the normal state of those innumerable abnormal conditions so often produced by the allopathic non-healing art, there is not and cannot be." Nor can it combat the extremely complicated and involved chronic miasmatic diseases of our era which have developed with the senseless and extravagant drugging applied by modern medicine with all its chemical sulphonamides and antibiotics.

Dr. Fredericka E. Gladwin had the following comment to make in connection with this method of Hahnemann: "We must remember that Hahnemann was still in the experimental stage of homoeopathy. He made tremendous progress from where he began in 1796 to where he left off in 1843, but since Hahnemann has left us there have been so many good homoeopaths experimenting...... that we should profit by their experience. I think that if Hahnemann could have lived until now, with the same experience that all these homoeopaths who have been between have had, and applied his remedies in very high potency, that he too would hold the application of one single potency until it gave out and then go higher, just as Kent and his followers have done with so much success."

Kent was the discoverer of the doctrine "Series in Degrees" which he foretold would become one of the most important subject in the treatment of chronic disease, and would lead to the development of a distinct class of prescribers in the school of Homoeopathy. To maintain the continuous curative action of the indicated remedy the doctrine of "Series in Degrees" must be understood and used. It is important to note that Hahnemann had no practical knowledge and experience of the action of those potencies which Kent used in accordance with his discovery. Fortunately both of the foregoing problems, namely the tackling of drug miasma and overcoming of the extremely complicated and involved chronic diseases of our era, are being, in certain fortunate cases, solved by physicians who faithfully follow Kent's method.

In the January 1886 edition of *The Homoeopathic Physician*, published by Lee, Kent called attention to the fact that Hahnemann's followers had been making progress since the death of the founder, citing the fact that although in Section 41 and 76 of the *Organon* Hahnemann had declared: "that certain diseases could not be eradicated as they had been complicated with drugs whose indications were only arbitrary and hypothetic," such diseases could in fact be wiped out and the drug symptoms subdued by very high attenuations. It must be pointed out that Hahnemann did not make any change in those two sections as regards the curability of drug miasma when he prepared the sixth edition of the *Organon* just before his death; it means that even after experimenting with "his last and most perfected method" he could not deal with this problem.

Kent's discovery has been verified consistently and his method found to be both efficacious and practicable. Like all of his good

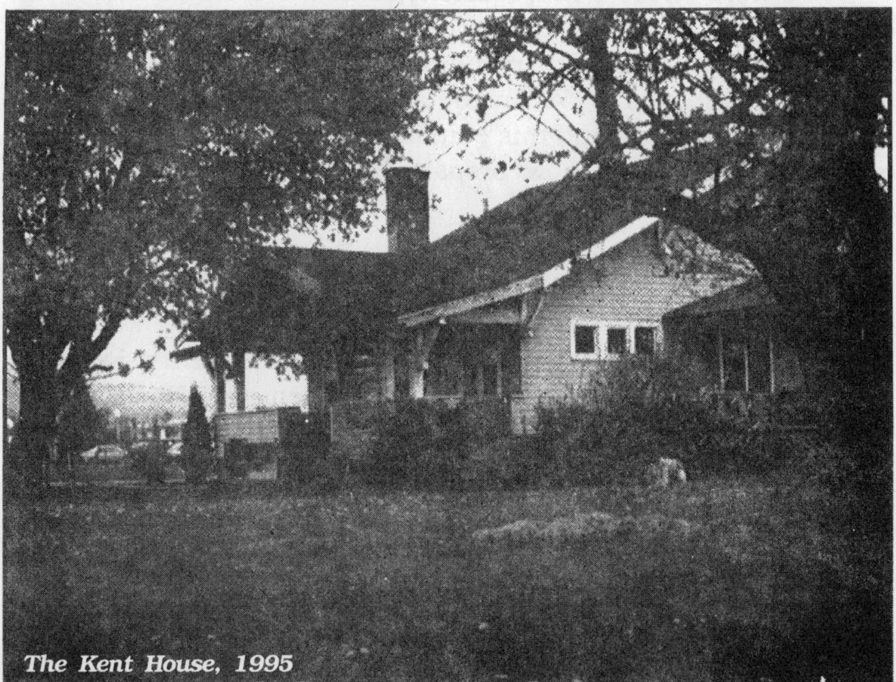

The Kent House, 1995

disciples I follow his procedure and have been doing so for some forty-seven years. It is also used by a number of our foremost physicians who are playing leading roles in the practice of the science and the art of homoeopathy and they, like myself, are carrying it out with the greatest satisfaction and praise it unreservedly. In the words of Dr. Gladwin: "Thanks to his untiring efforts and remarkable abilities, this past-master of the art and science of homoeo-pathic medicine has left us immortal works. More than that, he has shown us the example of infinite patience and unfailing kindness; he has guided our healing steps along the paths of homoeopathic truth, sparing neither time nor trouble to explain to us every stage of the journey ahead, constantly admonishing us and leading us back to the right road when, through ignorance, clumsiness or negligence we have strayed from the way of truth."

Kent was not pleased to learn that his students wanted to publish the stenographic notes which had been made of his lectures as he considered them insufficiently complete for the purpose he had in mind, but thanks to their insistence this work was revised by him and appeared in print, in 1990, under the title *Lectures on Homoeopathic Philosophy*.

This work exposes in a masterly form the theory and practice of the Hahnemannian doctrine. There have been several reprints of the *Philosophy* since 1900, including a memorial edition published in 1919. In the year 1958 I made a French translation of it, with many commentaries, and this edition was sold out within a month of publication : I am now preparing a second edition with an extensive and detailed index.

With reference to Kent's *Philosophy,* Dr. A. Grimmer, a student of Kent, says "that a full knowledge of it clarifies many of the obscure points in the *Organon* and enables the physician to have a deep perception of homoeopathic truths; to use Kent's *Repertory* expertly, it is necessary to have a complete knowledge of the contents of this book. This work has no equal in showing how to study the Materia Medica, grasp it fully and apply it successfully. For the homoeopath it is indispensable for it is the key which unlocks the storehouse of knowledge of homoeopathic healing. We must bear in mind that a single reading of the *Philosophy* will not suffice. It requires many careful perusals and much study to obtain a deep understanding of the truth of homoeopathy which it contains."

In the course of his lectures on Materia Medica Kent opened as a reference one of the ten volume of Hering's *Guiding Symptoms* and from this dry and analytical survey he created a lively synthesis and gave each remedy a distinct personality. He knew how to make the various elements of the picture, each with its lights and shades, stand out in all their originality.

I must mention that Hahnemann himself had written that there were many obscure and unreliable symptoms in our symptomatology. T.F. Allen (the author of the famous *Encyclopedia*) had also stressed the need of sifting our symptomatology because he said that the mistakes therein have been perpetuated from year to year. Hering had started collecting the reliable symptoms and Kent continued this work in the course of which he discovered that certain mistakes had been made by Hering. In addition to raising the grades of certain remedies in the *Guiding Symptoms* Kent has verified certain symptoms and has added a number of new ones; the very corrected copy of this book wherein Kent recorded his notes is now in my possession.

I would like to mention here some remarks made by Kent regarding Boenninghausen's famous *Repertory*. They were made in the July 1912 issue of the *Homoeopathician*. "There are books in existence that seem to foster the idea of pure Homoeopathy which have done much harm along with much good. Boenninghausen's *Therapeutic Pocket Book* has rendered all our old men a grand service, yet it is most defective and has caused many good men to shun repertories."

As he was unable to obtain a dictionary of symptoms sufficiently reliable for reference as to the remedies corresponding to a given symptom, he himself set about compiling a *Repertory of Symptoms*. In the course of this gigantic work he imposed a great strain on his health but the result was the best repertory ever made. At the outset he used as a guide the small work of C. Lippe, entitled *Repertory of the More Characteristic Symptoms of our Materia Medica* (published in New York in 1879) which was a repertory of some 318 pages, the ones of Jahr, Boenninghausen, Gentry, Biegler's diary and some pages of Minton's *Diseases of Women*. Kent's work was based on the principles of the *Organon* and when completed, it consisted of no less than 1,349 pages.

When the *Repertory* was at last ready some two hundred physicians placed an order for it, the price being $30 per copy. The cost for the mere setting of the print of this first edition amounted to $9,000 and Kent was somewhat discouraged to find that over half of those who had placed orders for it withdrew them at the last minute. Nevertheless, out of gratitude for what Homoeopathy had given to him and in the hope that it would be of use to homoeopathic profession, he decided to pay the required balance of $6,000 from his own pocket.

It was in 1897, after very many difficulties and at the cost of a great deal of eye strain for both Kent and his wife, that the *Repertory* was at last born. Kent still continued to collect notes and compile data, however, and in 1908 the second edition of the *Repertory* was published and Kent was still not satisfied. With some four hundred copies of the second edition still unsold, he started preparing the third edition and to this work he devoted the latter part of his life, unable, alas, to publish it while living. In 1914, two years before his death, he expressed concern about the completion of this third edition and remarked that neither he nor his wife would physically be able to read the proofs and he does not know who could. He had at that time become very frail but in spite of his failing health he was determined to continue. He would write for a short time and then rest, write again, then again take rest, until at last the work was finished. When he died in 1916 he left behind the completed third edition in manuscript form.

I would like to mention two pieces of advice which Kent would always give to his pupils, as they were transmitted to me by his most intimate disciples, Dr. Austin and Dr. Gladwin. They are:

1. "If you have prescribed a first remedy conscientiously and according to the homoeopathic doctrine, especially in an acute condition but also in chronic cases, and you get no result or unsatisfactory results, and if you go on to give a second and then a third, still with no effect, then, I beg you, stop, go no further. It is time to give placebo, which you might as well have done in the first place, and probably you would have gained considerable advantage by so doing. But it would certainly have been harder to apply this rule than, without sufficient accuracy but just in order to do something, to give one or two remedies of which you were uncertain, or which did not correspond to the essential symptoms of the case, either because you mistook the remedy or because you had not detected the symptoms of highest value. Never, therefore, prescribed

anything without having reconsidered the case. Like the stalker, waiting until the game is in his sights, wait patiently for the symptoms to develop before firing the bullet that will bring it down. Learn to *watch* and *wait*, and never lose your head."

2. "Whenever you examine a case with a view to determining the constitutional remedy, do not confine yourself to the Similimum alone, i.e. the remedy which bears especially the maximum qualitative similarity to the symptoms."

   This calls to mind the saga of the Swiss hero, Wilhelm Tell. When Tell was ordered by the landgrave to shoot an arrow at an apple placed on the head of his on, Tell laid an arrow to his cross-bow. He then took a second one from his quiver and hid it under his jerkin, so that, should his first arrow hit his son and not the apple, he might slay the man who had given the order with the reserve arrow. In the same way you should always have in reserve at least one alternative remedy — a *simile,* or what we today would call a *satellite* — as like as possible to the first, so that you will never be defenseless or at a loss for your second prescription.

DEMISE

Over worked with his teaching, his enormous practice requiring him to call on and receive many patients, his activities as a writer, an extensive correspondence as well as telegrams both by night and by day, asking without pause for his valued advice, he decided, at the insistence of his pupils, to have a rest and to take advantage of this respite at last to write a real book on Homoeopathy, as his two works, the *Philosphy* and *Materia Medica,* were regarded by him only as works of reference. Leaving his practice and his teaching

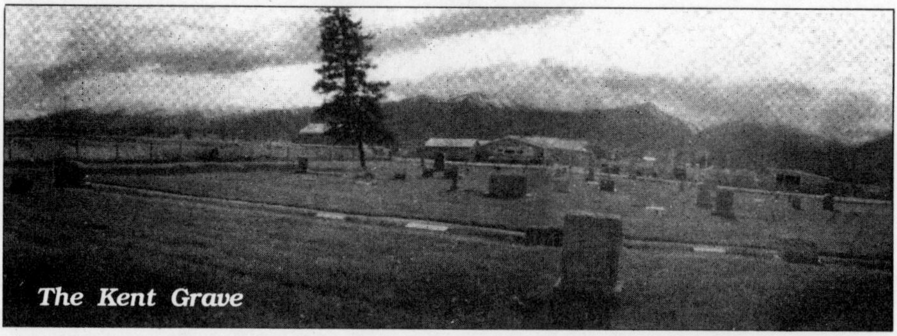

The Kent Grave

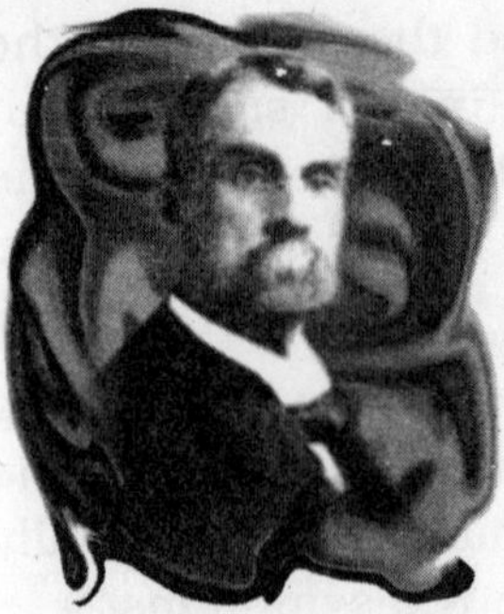

he went, now without difficulty, to his home in the country at Sunnyside Orchard in Stevensville in the State of Montana. But, alas, on his arrival the bronchial catarrh from which he had been suffering for some months was complicated by Bright's disease and after two weeks he succumbed, on June 6th, 1916. This was also due to the overwork which had completely worn him out over the years.

It was a terrible shock for the profession, for his friends, his innumerable patients and especially his many pupils to whom he had given so abundantly without concern for himself.

SECTION-L .... Page 185 to 188

L-1 ***Dr. Lilienthal, Samuel***
(Born: 05-12-1815 / Died: 03-10-1891) 186

Dr. Samuel Lilienthal

Born : 05-12-1815

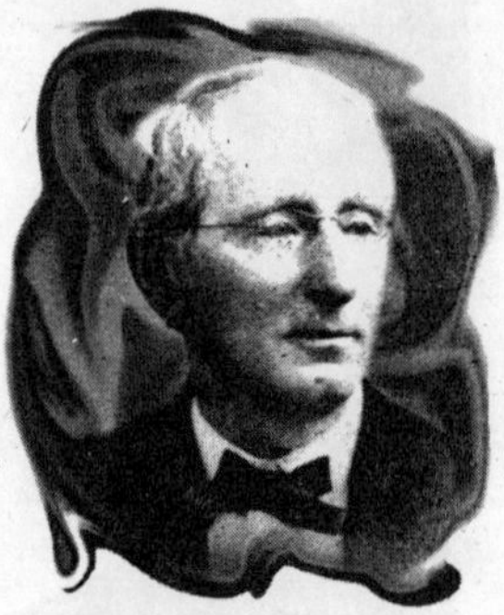

Died : 03-10-1891

BIRTH

Samuel Lilienthal was born in Munich, Germany, on the 5th of December, 1815.

EDUCATION

He passed his High School in 1834, and after passing from the University in the town and after a preparatory study of one year, he enrolled himself to study medicine. Samuel passed his "Doctor of Medicine" in 1838 and was attached to the Municipal Hospital at Munich until 1839 when he came to the United States of America.

PROFESSIONAL ACTIVITIES

In America, Dr. Lilienthal settled in Heidelberg, Pa, but after a short time went to South Carolina, where he remained until 1847 and finally came to the north and settled in Lockport, New York. He came in contact with a homoeopathic physician whose successful treatment of a case of scarlet fever and some other cases impressed him. He decided to study and practice homoeopathy. He left Lockport in 1850 and remained at Haverstraw, New York, for 7 years, ultimately shifting to New York City in 1857.

Through the influence of Dr. Constantine Hering he became the Associate Editor of THE NORTH AMERICAN JOURNAL OF HOMOEOPATHY and he conducted it alone for more than a decade, i.e., from 1873 to 1885. He had to resign from his favourite occupation because of his advancing years.

Dr. Lilienthal was also the co-editor of *American Homoeopathic Observer* from 1870 to 1885, and of *New York Journal of Homoeopathy*, 1874.

Section-L : Dr. Lilienthal, Samuel

When the New York Homoeopathic Medical College was opened, he entered the faculty in the chair of Clinical Medicine and Diseases of the Nervous System and remained on this position till 1886. When he left New York to spend the evening of his life with his family members in San Francisco, he was forced by his admirers to accept a Professorship at the Homoeopathic College in San Francisco but his old age soon compelled him to resign.

His sincerity and hard labors in the field of homoeopathic journalism are well-known. His journals became very famous. He translated articles from German, French, Spanish and Italian languages and wrote original articles and contributed articles for the prominent homoeopathic journals of his time. He was very regular and a popular face in the meetings of American Institute of Homoeopathy and State Society where his papers were highly appreciated.

He was a highly esteemed and respected practitioner and much soughtafter teacher.

His books HOMOEOPATHIC THERAPEUTICS & DISEASES OF THE SKIN are great contributions of everlasting value in homoeopathy.

DEMISE

He had suffered from recurrent attacks of angina pectoris due to atheroma of the coronary artery, and finally on saturday, the 3rd of October, 1891, at 1 A.M. he breathed his last.

His parting words to the readers of his journal were, "My mission is fulfilled. Perhaps this last lay of an old worker will touch a chord, and stir some physician up to do their duty, as literary work is most pleasant work........ Good bye; God bless you, my old readers."

HIS WRITINGS

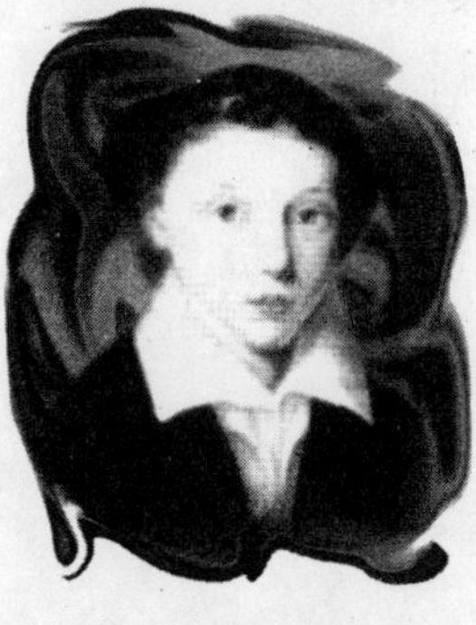

1873 : Characteristics of the New American Remedies.

1875 : Valedictory Address at the Commen-cement Exercises, March 4, 1875. Published by request of the Graduating Class of the New York Homoeopathic Medical College. 8 Volumes PP. 7. (Published with the Announce-ment for 1875-76).

1876 : A Treatise on Diseases of the Skin, P. 495.

(This was originally published as a monthly appendix to the Hahnemannian Monthly, 1874-76).

1878 : Homoeopathic Therapeutics. Boericke & Tafel. PP. 710.

1879 : The same, 2nd Edition, 8 Volume, PP. 835. (First edition was mostly burned at a fire at the bindery).

1890 : The same, 3rd, re-written and enlarged edition. PP. 1154.

1886 : Works on Materia Medica issued by Hahnemann, their Composition and Value. 8 Vo., PP. 39. (Reprint from Transactions of American Institute of Homoeopathy).

: Hereditary Insanity. Read before the American Institute of Homoeopathy at its late session held at Saratoga Springs, New York Pittsburgh. PP. 10. (Reprint from Transactions).

1887 : Etiology of Tuberculosis. (Reprint from Transactions of American Institute of Homoeopathy, 1886).

Translated Hildebrandt's Catarrh of Female Sexual Organs; Buchner's Morbus Brighti; Hahnemann's Geist der Homoeopathischen Heil-lehre.

SOURCE

1. Bradford, T.L. : Bibliography.
2. The Hahnemannian Monthly, (Volume XXVI), November 1891, P. 793.

SECTION-M .... Page 189 to 206

M-1 ***Dr. Majumdar, Jitendra Nath***
(Died: 30-11-1943) 190

M-2 ***Dr. Majumdar, Jnanendra Nath***
(Died: 15-09-1907 / Died: 29-11-1978) 191

M-3 ***Dr. Majumdar, Pratap Chandra***
(Died: 22-10-1922) 201

M-4 ***Dr. Mathur, K.N.***
(Born: 1906 / Died: 1977) 202

M-5 ***Dr. Mukherjee, A.N.***
(Died: 15-01-1954) 203

M-6 ***Dr. Mukherjee, Barid Baran***
(Born: 1873 / Died: 26-10-1940) 204

M-7 ***Dr. Muller, Father***
(Born: 13-03-1841 / Died: 01-11-1910) 205

M-8 ***Dr. Murty, V.R.***
(Born: 20-10-1904 / Died: 26-10-1940) 206

Dr. Jitendra Nath Majumdar

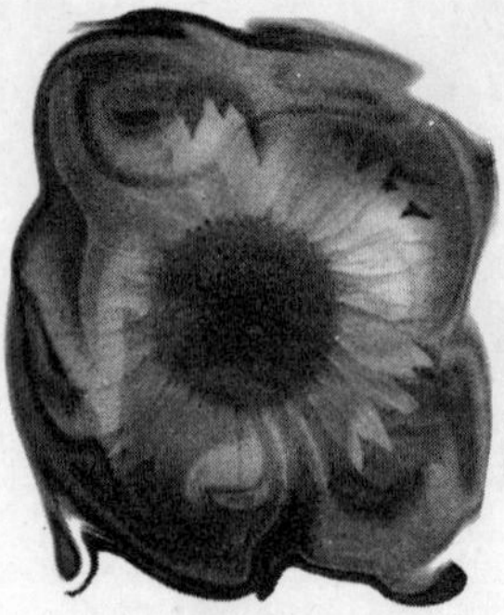

Died : 30-11-1943

Dr. Jitendra Nath Majumdar, M.D., the most illustrious and able son of Dr. Pratap Chandra Majumdar advanced the mission of his father until his demise on November 30, 1943. He was the President of 2nd All India Homoeopathic Conference at Gaya. He was the founder of the Pratap Chandra Memorial Homoeopathic Medical College and Hospital, which later turned into Pratap and Hering Memorial Homoeopathic Medical College and Hospital. He is the proud father of Indian homoeopath, Dr. Jnanendra Nath Majumdar.

Dr. Jnanendra Nath Majumdar

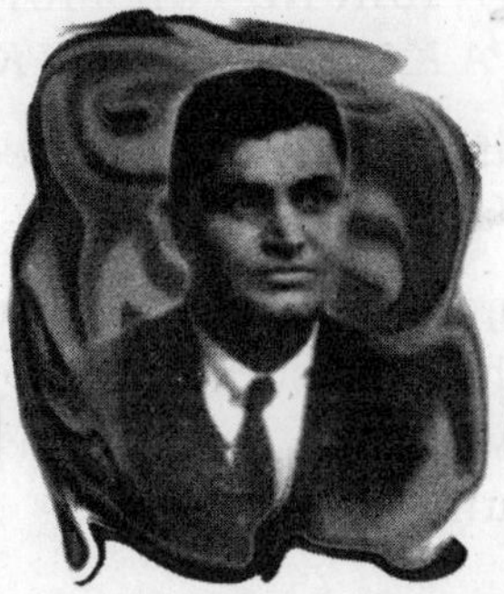

Born : 15-09-1907 Died : 29-11-1978

NATIONAL POET DINKAR WROTE

"JAI HO JAG ME JALE JAHAN BHI NAMAN PUNIT ANAL KO
JIS NAR MEN BHI BASE HAMARA NAMAN TAJ KO, BAL KO"

"Our salutations to the great light, where ever it is lit; Our salutations to the greatness, to dynamism in whomsoever it manifest."

What an apt preface for the story of the life and the deeds of the great personality, the dynamic leader, the learned teacher, the successful physician, the devoted homoeopath, the kindhearted man, the stead fast fighter for the oppressed and the neglected, be it human beings, be it the healing art of homoeopathy. We salute him, his hollowed memory and we feel proud that he belonged to us in life and he belongs to us in death, we honour him because he guided us while living and left us a blean path to follow when he is no more.

Homoeopathic history is full of men and women who were educated and learned, intelligent and wise, dedicated and devoted, successful and famous, talented and dynamic yet the history and life of Dr. Jnan Majumdar, as he was commonly referred to, is unique and unsurpassable in respect to homoeopathic back ground of family, general and medical education, academic excellence, social influence, legislative achievements, successful practice, acid tongue, lotus heart and service to the poor people, an arrogant exterior, a stoic interior and, over and above everything, an uncommon metamorphosis of dialectic materialism, progressive views, homoeopathic philosophy and Hindu Vedantism. In any one of these branches of human knowledge and achievement there were homoeopaths who could out-class and supercede him, but taken all together only one individual had all these and more than any one in homoeopathic history, it was Dr. J.N. Majumdar.

Tulsidas, the author of Ramcharit Manas RAMAYANA said,

"KAVITA KAR KE TULSI NA LASE,
LASI PA KAVITA TULSI KI KALA".

"It was not Tulsidas who was benefitted by poetry, but it was poetry which was enriched by Tulsi."

It was not Jnan Majumdar who benefitted by homoeopathy but it was homoeopathy which was enriched by Majumdar, and thus we always think the two to be same and inseparable, Dr. Jnan Majumdar & homoeopathy.

ANCESTORS & FAMILY

In India, Dr. Majumdar's family and ancestors were one of the earliest perceptors and torch bearers of homoeopathy and remained a forceful current of the stream of homoeopathy. The flame which was lit by Dr. Bihari Lal Bhaduri acquired glorious brilliance through the efforts and labors of his son-in-law Dr. Pratap Chandra Majumdar whose son Dr. Jitendra Nath Majumdar carried the torch of homoeopathy further and with enhanced glory.

The seed of the tree of homoeopathic family to which Dr. Majumdar belonged was put by Dr. Bihari Lal Bhaduri, who was born at Santragachi, in Howrah district in 1840, was married to Nrityakali, the daughter of a famous Jamindar Ram Das Goswami of Shree Rampur, passed L.M.S. from Medical College and served in the states of Orissa and Bihar as a Government Medical Officer, came in close contact with Dr. Salzer and Rajendra Dutta and after observing some miracles by homoeopathy converted to homoeopathy and earned high acclaim as a homoeopathic physician, author and early stalwart of homoeopathy in India.

His sons Dr. Aghor Charan and Dr. Birendra Lal were homoeopathic physicians. His eldest daughter Barahini Devi was married to Dr. Pratap Chandra Majumdar, the son of Krishna Jiban Majumdar and Ranga Devi of Chatra village in Nadia district, who proved to be the greatest pioneer of homoeopathy in India. Pratap Chandra Majumdar, an allopathic physician converted to homoeopathy was instrumental in establishing the first homoeopathic institution, Calcutta Homoeopathic Medical School, later College, in India and was Founder Editor of INDIAN HOMOEOPATHIC REVIEW and a renowed author. He proved many Indian drugs which were included in the books of Materia Medica of Clarke, Allen and Boericke, S.C. Ghosh, etc. His second son Khagendra Nath, a Barrister and the Secretary of Bengal Legislative Council, after his retirement became the Honorary Registrar of the newly established Homoeopathic Faculty in this state. His third son Nagendra Nath passed M.D. from America and became a renowned homoeopath. All of his 10 daughters were highly educated which in itself was a courageous act in those days. His eldest daughter Surbala was married to the famous Bengali poet and dramatist Dwijendra Lal Roy of Krishnanagar and the proud mother of Dilip Roy, the famous artist, while the fifth daughter Swarnalata was married to Dr. N.M. Chowdhury, renowned homoeopathic author, founder-Editor of HOME & HOMOEOPATHY and the founder-Principal of Bengal Allen Homoeopathic College.

Pratap Majumdar's eldest son Jitendra Nath Majumdar was born in Calcutta on tuesday, 4th July, 1876 finished his early education under Pandit Ishwar Chandra Vidyasagar in Metropolitan School and joined the Presidency College after passing the entrance examination; he left for U.S.A. and received his M.D. from Chicago Hahnemann Medical College; he was very close to Dr. Allen. In 1903 he married Smt. Rajeswari Devi. Jiten Babu remained a voracious reader till the end of his earthly life, he had a vast collection of books and journals on homoeopathy and general medicine. Since homoeopathy was not a recognised system of treatment then and the British Government was not willing to heed to a homoeopath, tenacious Jitendra Nath at the age of 44 years took admission into Campbell, present Nil Ratal Sarkar Medical College and Hospital, and passed allopathic L.M.F. examination. He was the Honorary Secretary of Calcutta Homoeopathic Medical College and later on established Pratap Chandra Memorial Homoeopathic Medical College and aslo established a homoeopathic hospital at Madhupur in Bihar. Dr. Jitendra Nath Majumdar and his kind hearted wife Smt. Rajeshwari Devi were the proud parents of two daughters, namely Shibani Majumdar nee Chakraborty and Bharati Majumdar nee Bhattacharya and six sons, namely Dr. Pratul Chandra Majumdar. Dr. Jnanendra Nath Majumdar, Dr. Atul Chandra Majumdar, Dr. Rajendra Nath Majumdar, Dev Kumar Majumdar and the one who died at an early age.

BIRTH & EDUCATION

Jnan Majumdar, the second son of Dr. Jitendra Nath Majumdar, was born on sunday, the 15th of September, 1907.

He was a student of the reputed Metropolitan School, where Swami Vivekananda was once a teacher. He passed matriculate examination in 1922 and passed intermediate science in 1924 from City College of Calcutta. He passed his M.B.B.S. examination, in 1929 with Honours in Surgery and Midwifery, passed M.Sc., in 1932 L.R.C.P.C. from London in 1933 and received his F.R.C.S. in 1937 from Edinburgh University. Then in 1957 he passed the D.M.S. examination in Homoeopathy from West Bengal, and in 1973 was awarded M.D. from the Council of Homoeopathic Medicine, West Bengal.

His childhood was spent in a wholesome homoeopathic family and in an atmosphere of education, enlightenment and progressive views and in a circle of celebrities.

RELIGIOUS INCLINATIONS

He was an Indian Communist in the true sense, progressive, free from all religious superstitions but in very personal life a disciple of Bharat Maharaj.

DR. MAJUMDAR & HOMOEOPATHY

Dr. Majumdar, born in a homoeopathic family of three generations had seen the miracles and limitations of homoeopathy from his childhood. Homoeopathy was in his blood and bones. His highest education in allopathic surgery and medicine, master's degree in physiology, deep knowledge of history of medicine and homoeopathic philosophy has made his position unique in the history of homoeopathy, and this honour and record will ever remain unchallenged. The combination of all the above said factors had given him a very clear vision of the scope and limitations of homoeopathy, and complete freedom from the blind faith and oracle-worshipping tendencies of ignorant homoeopaths and in true sense was a practitioner of classic and perfect homoeopathy.

He was an admirer of Kent, Boericke, Stuart Close, but usually preferred Boenninghausen's methods and books in daily practice. It was Boennighausen and Boger whom he held in highest esteem and followed in difficult and typical cases.

In addition to it, he had developed a keen insight into the physiognomical studies of medicines and, at times, was able to prescribe medicines easily on the basis of the physiognomy, phrenological character and external appearance of the patients.

Another aspect of his homoeopathic character was that he never stopped the experiments and was constantly verifying and experimenting with the proved as well as the clinical characteristics of the remedies.

His fame as a successful physician not only touched the last boundaries of this country but patients used to consult him in person and by correspondence from the neighbouring countries like Nepal, Sri Lanka, East Pakistan and from far off places like Russia, Canada, America, etc.

Dr. Majumdar, his friends and family played a great role in the enactment of the statutes of State Faculty in 1943 and a very vital and decisive role in the enactment of Homoeopathic Act of 1963.

The syllabus of Homeopathic Council which was followed as a model throughout India and neighbouring countries was the brain-child of Dr. Majumdar.

In the Draft Act for Central Council of Homoeopathy the influence, labors and expenses of Dr. Majumdar were supreme and greatest.

Even from his sick bed he sent a letter on 2.9.1975 to Mr. S.N. Sen the Vice-Chancellor, University of Calcutta outlining the dangers of the haste and hurry with which affiliation was granted to the four homoeopathic colleges, without formulating curriculum and before the Government take over of the hospitals. He wrote "I want to see homoeopathy in its proper form than the glamours of University, which has spoiled homoeopathy in other parts of the world." What a prevision! What prophetic words!

His understanding and the devotion to pure homoeopathy can be seen in that he himself being an allopathic convert wrote to Dr. P.K. Bose, Pro-vice chancellor of Calcutta University, "Inspecting body...... should see that senior qualified homoeopaths like D.M.S. (Cal.) are in charge of their hospital........ converted homoeopaths with allopathic qualifications should strictly be avoided.........". All that he feared and wanted to avoid is happening to homoeopathic colleges, hospitals and homoeopathy. The short-sighted leaders of the profession did not hear to the most qualified, wise and sane voice and are now repenting their deeds.

He must have felt contented that he was involved in the legislation of Homoeopathic Acts for the state and the nation.

The shadow of this great tree and the light of his knowledge was evident in anything which happened in homoeopathy in the state or national level although in many instances it was not discernible.

He must have wept the tears of pleasure and achievement when his dream came true and Central Homoeopathy Council Act was passed and National Institute of Homoeopathy was started in Calcutta.

He was aware of the hypocrisy and learned pretensions of the senior homoeopathic physicians and teachers and so his wise advice to younger physicians was "WHEN ALWAYS IN DIFFICULTY, GO TO THE FOUNTAIN HEAD, YOU ARE YOUR BEST CONSULTANT."

The Majumdars ruled the homoeopathic world through their dispensaries and offices spread in the South, North, East and West of Calcutta, viz. 3 Chorwringhee Square (95E, Central Avenue), 29, Strand Road, 203/1, Cornwallis Street, 34, Theatre Road, 162, Russa Road, 14/1, Narkeldanga North Road, and in this dynasty of homoeopathic saints, savants and kings Jnanendra Nath was most distinguished in education, influence, practice, status, glory and fame. About him, Dr. Sudhir Adhirari wrote, "This physician of opulence and glory is, in a nutshell, an Emperor of Bengal," Dr. Adhirari would have been more correct had he said India, instead of Bengal.

But inspite of his international fame, national name and enviable success the communist, the Vedantist Jnan Majumdar said "I HAVE TRIED MY BEST TO PLAY A GOOD INNINGS ASSOCIATING MYSELF WITH THE SUFFERINGS, NEEDS AND PROBLEMS OF MY PATIENTS. LIFE HAS TAUGHT ME NOT TO GIVE UP OR DESPAIR BUT TO KEEP ONE'S CHIN UP. THERE CAN BE NO GREATER REWARD THAN SERVING THE PEOPLE ALTHOUGH I REMEMBER MY FAILURES MORE THAN MY SUCCESSES."

ACADEMIC ATTACHMENTS

He was a Member of:

State Faculty of Homoeopathic Medicine; West Bengal.

Homoeopathic Enquiry Committees.

Homoeopathic Advisory Committee (1956 to 1966).

Homoeopathic Research Sub-Committee since 1958.

Health Panel, Planning Commission.

EDUCATIONAL ATTACHMENTS

Served as a visiting Professor in Surgery in National Medical School (later College).

And was Principal of Pratap Hering Memorial Homoeopathic College.

POLITICAL ATTACHMENTS

Although he was not thoroughly involved but he was a member of Communist Party of India. He was elected as a member to Legislative Assembly.

PROFESSIONAL ATTACHMENTS

He was actively associated in different positions with Bengal Homoeopathic Institution, and was the President of All India Homoeopathic Medical Association, attended International Congress and was the chief support and spirit behind All India Conferences held in Calcutta.

In 1951 he presided over the first session of Assam State Homoeopathic Conference at Silchar.

DRUG PROVING

He discovered and made extensive experiments with Aqua cosmos.

LITERARY CONTRIBUTIONS

This is a very incomplete list of the writings of Dr. Majumdar because many of the articles could not be traced. The later issues of Indian Homoeopathic Review contain many articles by him.

1. Chronic Amoebiasis : Souvenir in memorium of J.N. Majumdar, 1979, P. 31.
2. How to study Materia Medica: Souvenir of West Bangal State Homoeopathic Conference, 1971.
3. Pratap Chandra Majumdar (Bangla), ibid. P. 35.
4. Teaching in homoeopathic institutions on an undergraduate basis.

   It gave complete division of aphorisms of organon on the basis of contents and became a ready reckoner for homoeopathic teachers and students.

5. As an Associate Editor of Indian Homoeopathic Review he contributed articles.
6. Homoeopathy, Surgery & Pathology.
7. Prognostic value of Similimum.
8. Carbuncle.

DEMISE

The great Hindi Saint poet Kabir Das said,

"AYE HAIN SO JAYENGE RAJA, RUNK, FAKIR;
EK SINHASAN CHADHI CHALE, EK BANDHE JANJIR"

Whoever has come, will go, be it the king, the pauper, the beggar.

But some go back riding a throne while some go sackled in chains.

His wide practice, social, political, homoeopathic and other engagements were enough to break an iron constitution. He was unable to take care of his health and self and he suffered a wild heart attack and was bedridden. But just after a few days the crowd of his students, professional colleagues, self-seekers and his patients thronged again. Although the hours became regular, habits modulated, visitors screened but Dr. Majumdar was too courageous and dutiful to care for himself. Besides, it was too late and the cruel hands of unkind death struck again. This time fatally, seriously and finally. On the 29th of November, 1978 his heart refused to carry the load of the physical and mental activities of an intellectual giant, and educationist, a crusader, a world famous physician and a legislator belonging to a political faith which has avowed aim of protecting the down-trodden and have-nots, a born rebel who moved ahead of time and stood always on the front of progress and advancement. After the highest academic and allopathic medical education and employment in an institution, he converted to homoeopathy, in a Congress-party-ruled nation he became a communist.

India was the target of a popular uproar at the time of Chinese aggression in 1962 he went to the side of break away C.P.I. (M) and when the leftists were waiting in the wings of power his inclinations were towards the ultra-left.

And when on 29th of November, 1978 at 12-15 P.M. the Homoeopathic Emperor left this world to go to the place of ancestors and predecessors, to the land of no-return, it was a significant coincidence that it was a Wednesday. Wednesday is the day of the WODEN, the chief deity of Norse mythology, a storm-God and worshipped chiefly by the warrior nobles and receiver of the souls at Valhalla, which is the abode of warriors who go out daily to wage wars and return at nightfall to feast with WODEN. And our warrior Dr. Majumdar, battles daily not through his body, but through his spirit and teaching to us, against diseases, death and sufferings, feeling proud when we are successful as physicians and sad when we fail to heal. That fateful day when Dr. Majumdar breathed his last homoeopathy lost a fearless experimenter, fighter and the most educated homoeopath of the world; it lost the voice, the pen which was respected, feared and seldom contradicted; it lost the only physician who could talk to politicians as their better, to the bureaucrats as a legislator, to the law-enacting legislative Assembly as a member, to the errant homoeopaths as a confessor and guide, to the true homoeopaths as a symbol of success, to the students as the height to which homoeopathy can take them.

Majumdar's death was the end of a golden era in homoeopathy. It was the end of the head of the homoeopathic clan of Bhaduries & Majumdars. It was the drop-scene of the domination of classical homoeopathy.

It was the cessation of only one mind in India, nay world, which could judge best the line of treatment, need, and prognosis of a patient. Few only could have realised that on the fateful day passed away a homoeopath whose academic qualifications were highest in the history of homoeopathy.

HIS FAMILY & CHILDREN

All his sons and daughters are highly educated and well settled as surgeons and engineers. The delicately built, calm, educated and beautiful youngest daughter is the flagbearer of the family profession and tradition of medicine, homoeopathic medicine. She is the figure behind Majumder Pharmacy which has a name for supplying the profession with pure and genuine medicines.

Judging from the busy life of Dr. Majumdar and his multiferous and multifaceted activities and engagements one wonders who was the force behind the scene who brought and order and discipline in his hectic activities, who looked after the education and upbringing of the children, who kept the house in order and then it is not difficult to figure out the strong-willed, kind-hearted disciplinarian Smt. Anima Majumdar who was 'the great woman' behind this 'great man'. Dr. Majumdar's wife, Anima Majumdar, has worked in silence and had received no glory, has remained a solid and powerful anchor of the family, the tradition, the children, the clan of the immortal families of Bhaduries, Majumdars, Rays, Chowdhuries. The Emperor ruled the homoeopathic world, this self-denying lady looked after the home and when the emperor has gone, the empire is going away, the empress remains, the last symbol and the last link of a great tradition, a great era of famous, successful, and deathless family of homoeopathic Majumdars.

SOURCE MATERIALS

1. Hahnemann (Bangla), Magh, 1385, Volume 61, No. 9.
2. Homoeopathic Bijnan Parisad, Souvenir, May, 1989.
3. South Calcutta Co-ordination Committee, Homoeopathic Medical Association of India & Citizens of South Calcutta week-round ceremony on the occasion of 224 years Birth Anniversary of Dr. S. Hahnemann & in memorium of Dr. J.N. Majumdar, 1979.
4. The Homoeopathic Sandesh, April, 1970.
5. The Homoeopathic Sandesh, Auditorial, April, 1970.
6. Chikitshak Samaj Patrika, 1969, Volume 1, No. 1.
7. Amrita Bazar Patrika, 5th December, 1977.
8. Hahnemannian Gleanings, July, 1951 (Vol. XVIII, No. 7).
9. Souvenir, West Bengal State D.M.S. conference, 1969.

Dr. Pratap Chandra Majumdar

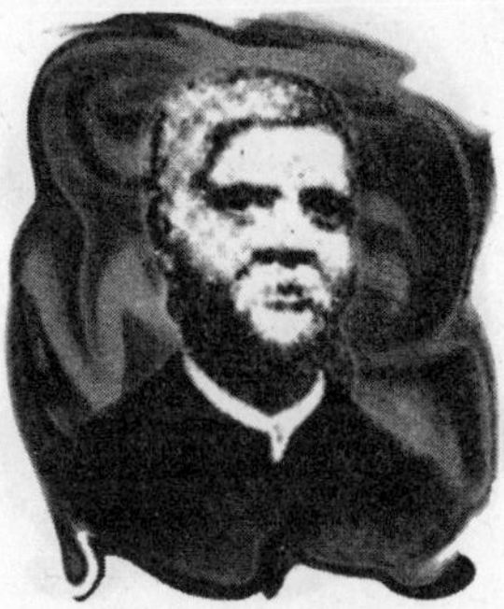

Died : 22-10-1922

Dr. Pratap Chandra Majumdar took L.M.S. degree from Calcutta Medical College in 1878 and later got honorary degree of M.D. from U.S.A. He was converted to homoeopathy by his father-in-law, Dr. B.L. Bhaduri. He fortified his grasp on Hahnemannian homoeopathy as the worthy assistant to Dr. L. Salzer for pretty long time. Later, he amassed immense fortune simply by the practice of homoeopathy. He expired on October 22, 1922, leaving behind not only huge wealth and properties, but also two successive generations of gems in the homoeopathic field.

He proved a number of indigenous drugs, wrote large number of books in English and Bengali which still inspire thousands of homoeopaths. He edited the Indian Homoeopathic Review, the second oldest homoeopathic journal in India, after Dr. Mahendra Lal Sircar's Calcutta Homoeopathic Journal. He attended the Fourth International Homoeopathic Congress held in Chicago in June 1891. In collaboration with Dr. D.N. Roy he established the Calcutta Homoeopathic Medical College in 1881 and maintained it till his death.

Dr. K.N. Mathur

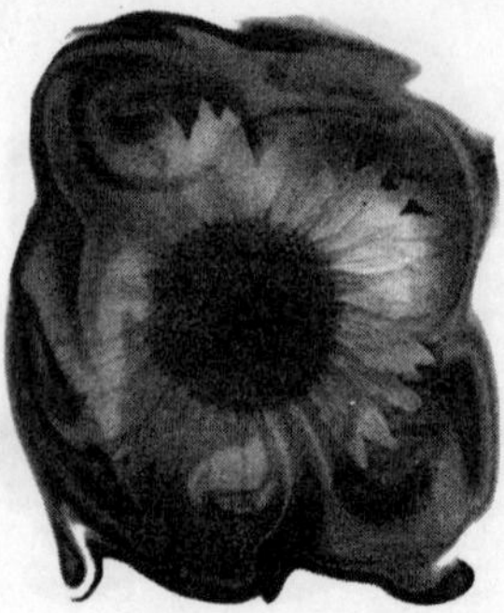

Born : 1906 Died : 1977

On April 10, 1906, a great homoeopath was bon at Allahabad in the family of educationists, doctors and a highly cultured family of Mathur Kayastha; he was Dr. K. N. Mathur (Kailash Narain Mathur) M.B., B.S., M.F. Hom. (London).

He took his M.B., B.S. degree from Lucknow Medical College in the year 1933. At the call of the nation during the World War-II he joined the emergency Military Commission in 1939 and continued to serve the army till 1948.

He worked ceaselessly for promoting homoeopathic understanding, its uplift and for its due recognition from the Govt. As Secretary of the Delhi Homoeopathic Medical Association for 10 years, he organised meetings and sought interviews with proper Govt. authorities, including the President of India.

In the year 1958, he went of England and did his M. F. Hom. On retuning to India in 1960 he joined the A.H. Medical College, Kottayam in Kerala as Professor of Pathology and Medicine. After 5 years with College, at the call of Dr. Yudhvir Singh, he came back to Delhi and organised Nehru Homoeopathic College and Hospital at Defence Colony, New Delhi.

He was the author of the following books : 1. Diabetes Mellitus, 2. Organon, 3. Repertory, 4. Pathology, 5. Systematic Materia Media, 6. Principles of Prescribing.

He died on January 28, 1977, due to sudden heart failure.

Section-M : Dr. Mathur, K. N.

Dr. A.N. Mukherjee

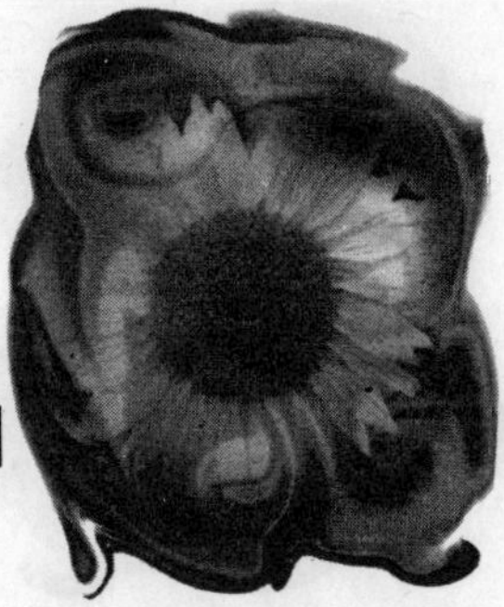

Died : 15-01-1954

Dr. A. N. Mukherjee, M.D., one of the most respected homoeopaths of Culcutta, expired on January 15, 1954. He along with Dr. Jitendra Nath Majumdar and many others fought strenuously for and ultimately brought into existence the General Council and State Faculty of Homoeopathic Medicine, Bengal, on April 1, 1943 and belonged to the first batch of its members.

Dr. Barid Baran Mukherjee

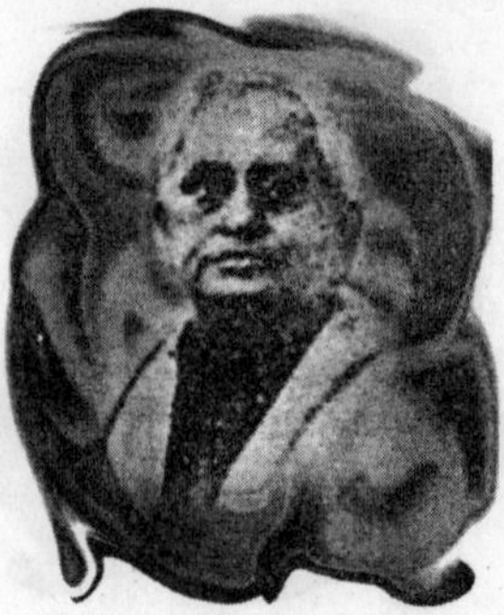

Born : 1873 **Died : 26-10-1940**

Dr. Barid Baran Mukherjee, L.M.S., who was one of the ablest, noblest and most respected homoeopaths of Calcutta, expired on October 26, 1940 at the age of 67.

Dr. Father Mueller

Born : 13-03-1841

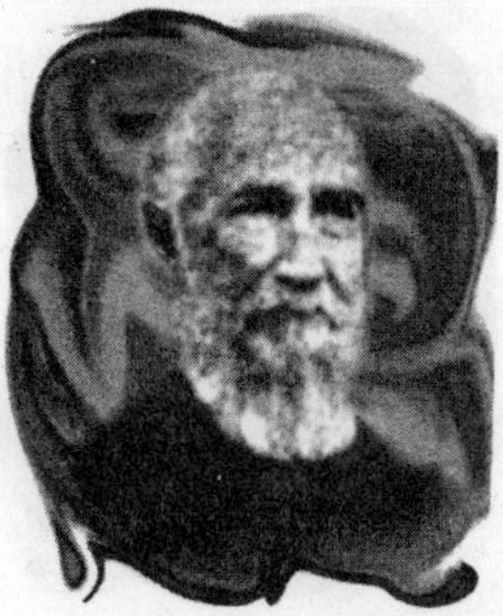

Died : 01-11-1910

Father Mueller was born at Westphalia in Germany on March 13, 1841. He suffered from various ailments, which baffled the skill of the allopathic physicians. He was thus compelled to have recourse to homoeopathy, and by the help of this system he recovered his health. With the noble object of relieving the sufferings of others he took up seriously the study of homoeopathy in U.S.A. and France and acquired proficiency in it.

He came to Mangalore (South India), on December 31, 1878, as a member of the first group of Jesuit missionaries and brought with him a small chest of homoeopathic medicines. With these he treated the students and others who came to him for medical aid. He opened the Homoeopthic Poor Dispensary at Kanakanady, Mangalore in 1880.

In 1897, Fr. Mueller received the secret formula of the Socleri-Bellotti Specifics from the Father General of the Society of Jessus. These are now known as Fr. Mueller's Specifics all over India and abroad.

In 1891, he started the St. Josph's Leprosy Hospital and Asylum to house and treat the poor and abandoned leprosy patients of the Mangalore and South Kanara Districts.

In 1895, he started building up a General Hospital. Even in the midst of all this work, building up, expansion and devoted service of the sick, Fr. Mueller found time for writing and publishing many useful books on homoeopathy and the tissue remedies.

Early in 1910, he was attacked by asthma, which brought on cardiac trouble and on November 1, 1910 he passed away peacefully.

Section-M : Dr. Mueller, Father

Dr. V.R. Murty

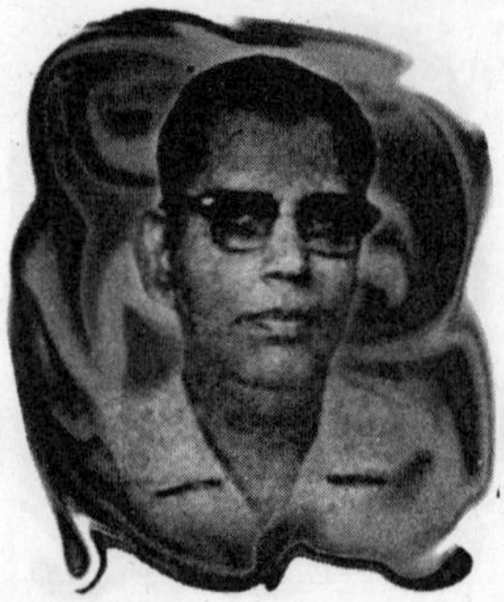

Born : 20-10-1904 **Died : 26-10-1940**

Dr. V.R. Murty, a pioneer of homoeopathy in the south and founder-architect of the Indian Institute of Homoeopaths and Bahola Group Concerns, was born in a village near Tiruvarus on October 20, 1904.

Even when he was very young, it was his ambition to become a doctor and serve the sick and the suffering. But his financial conditions did not permit him to join a medical college.

He proceeded to Bombay where one of his sisters got a violent attack of pneumonia complicated with peritonitis. Since allopathic doctors were not hopeful about her recovery, on the advise of one of his friends, she was administered homoeopathic medicines and she got well. Consequently, he become interested in the homoeopathic science and went on reading books on it.

In 1939, he founded the Indian Institute of Homoeopaths. To cater to the needs of the practicing students and to make available standard homoeopathic medicines at a reasonable cost to the homoeopathic profession and the public at large, he started a Pharmaceutical Laboratory manned by qualified personnel. Today the institute functions with its own research and clinical laboratories, out-patient and in-patient hospitals, and a factory manufacturing medicines to accurate standards.

In token of his meritorious service for the cause of homoeopathy, he was awarded the title 'Homoeopathic Chikitsa Acharya' (H.C.A.) by Dr. Swami Sivananda of the Yoga Vedanta, Forest University, Rishikesh, and D.H.O.M. Diploma by the Registrar of Homoeopathic Practitioners, England.

Dr. V.R. Murty was an able physician and had treated successfully a number of cases declared hopeless by others. He propagated the science of homoeopathy as widely as possible and his demise is no doubt a great loss to homoeopathy in India.

Section-M : Dr. Murty, V.R.

SECTION-N .... Page 207 to 209

N-1 ***Dr. Nash, Eugene Beuharis***
(Born: 08-03-1838 / Died: 06-11-1917) 208

N-2 ***Dr. Nag, S.K.***
(Died: 22-03-1937) 209

Dr. Eugene Beuharis Nash

Born : 08-03-1838

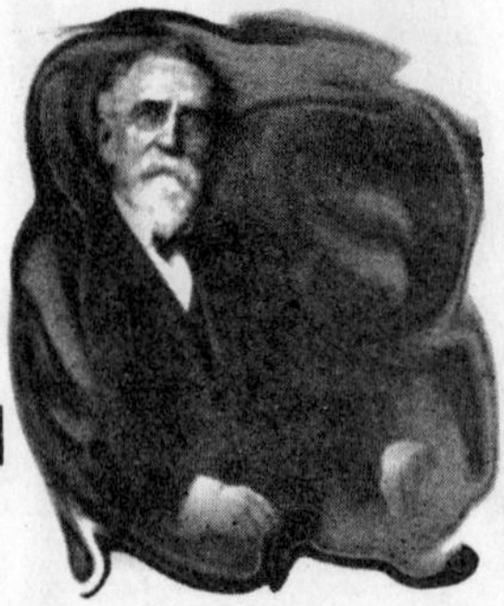

Died : 06-11-1917

Dr. E.B. Nash, M.D., was born on the 8th of March, 1838. He studied medicine with Dr. T.L. Brown in Binghamton, New York. In 1874, he graduated from Cleveland Homoeopathic College. He set up his practice in Cortland, New York. He was professor of materia medica for seven years at the New York Homoeopathic Medical College. In 1903 he was the president of the International Hahnemannian Association. He also gave lectures at the Homoeopathic Hospital in London, in 1905.

Nash wrote, *"Leaders in Homoeopathic Therapeutics"*, a brief book on materia medica. Upon the 4th edition, in 1913, of his book, "Leaders in Homoeopathic Therapeutics", Nash wrote: "To my good wife, who has done the clerical work under my dictation, is due much praise. This on account of my blindness. As I draw near the end of my earthly career I hope to leave an influence for good that will live many years."

He died on the 6th of November, 1917.

Dr. S.K. Nag

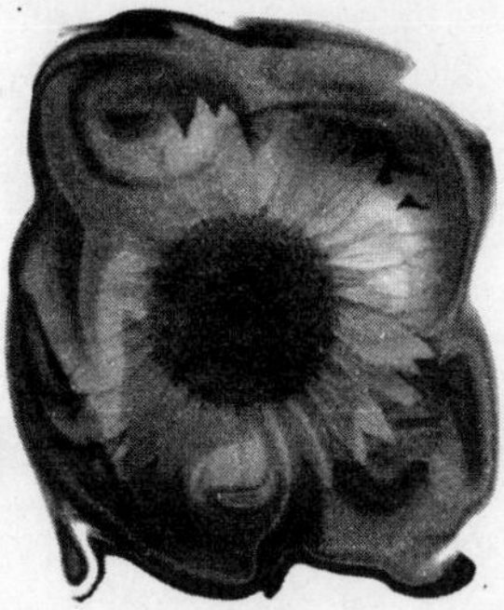

Died : 22-03-1937

Dr. S. K. Nag, L.M.S., M.D., was not only a great homoeopath but also a great teacher. He was the Secretary of the Calcutta Homoeopathic Medical College after the demise of the founder-secretary, Dr. D.N. Ray. He expired on March 22, 1937.

Enjoy, don't regret, the effort required to achieve success.

SECTION-P

SECTION-P .... Page 211 to 212

P-1 Dr. Pillai, M.N.
(Born: 04-04-1882 / Died: 1942) 212

Dr. M.N. Pillai

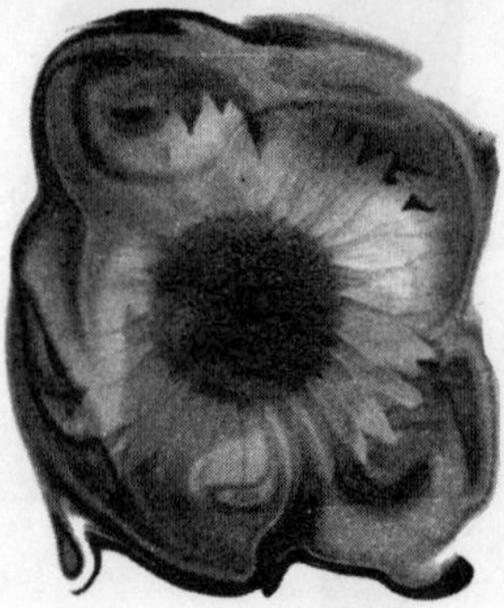

Born : 04-04-1882 Died : 1942

Dr. M.N. Pillai was born on April 4, 1882 at Trivandrum. He passed four years' course in homoeopathy from Calcutta and set up practice in Cochin just at the age of twenty-four.

Dr. Pillai's homoeopathic drugs were so effective that in the matter of cholera alone, he was nicknamed 'Cholera Doctor.' In the Legislature he worked for the recognition of homoeopathic system of medicine and establishment of homoeopathic dispensaries and hospitals by the Government.

On April 17, 1928, he piloted a resolution in the Legislative Assembly demanding recognition by the Government to the homoeopathic system of medicine which was passed with a great majority. His most important work was the publication of an exhaustive book in Malayalam, entitled *'What is Homoeopathy'*.

His ambition was the start free dispensaries and a nursing-home to give a new impetus to the cause of this system of medicine in his State. While he was working towards this end, his health deteriorated and he expired in March, 1942.

Section-P : Pillai, M.N.

SECTION-R .... Page 213 to 217

R-1 ***Dr. Roberts, Herbert A.***
(Born: 07-05-1868 / Died: 13-10-1950) 214

R-2 ***Dr. Roy, V.M. Kulkarni***
(Born: 1908 / Died: 07-11-1965) 217

Dr. Herbert A. Roberts

Born : 07-05-1868

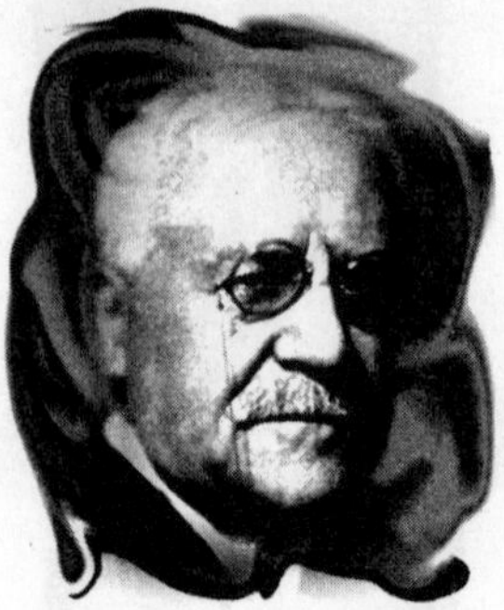

Died : 13-10-1950

Dr. Herbert A. Roberts is a well-known name in the world of homoeopathic philosophy. Over many years Dr. Roberts articles were universally popular and unanimously accepted and read for their scholarly exposition of the various sides of the homoeopathic philosophy and practice.

BIRTH & EARLY EDUCATION

Dr. Roberts was born on the 7th of May, 1868 in Riverton of Connecticut. For his primary education he was admitted in the Public School of Winsted. He completed his graduation in 1886 from Winsted High School.

MEDICAL EDUCATION

After completing his graduation Dr. Roberts decided to make his career in medicine, particularly in homoeopathy. With this object he took admission in New York Homoeopathic Medical College from where he did his matriculation in 1892. After matriculation he studied for four years more and obtained graduation in homoeopathic medicine, in 1896, from the same institution.

MEDICAL PRACTICE

Dr. Roberts started his medical practice in 1896, in Brattleboro in Vermont. He practiced here for three years as a successful practitioner.

Three years later he closed his clinic in Brattlebores and shifted to Shelton, Connecticut. He started his clinic here in

---

Section-R : Roberts, Herbert A.

Elizabeth Street at Deroy, Connecticut, just across the Housatonic River from Sheton. He practiced homoeopathy for nearly fifty years.

CONTRIBUTIONS

Dr. Roberts became a member of the Connecticut Homoeopathic Medical Society after starting his practice in Shelton. He became president of this society for 2 years, from 1904 to 1906. Later he was elected as its secretary and remained in this position for more than thirty years.

In 1907, he became member of American Institute of Homoeopathy. Dr. Roberts was elected to membership in the International Hahnemannian Association in the year 1910. He was entrusted with the Presidential post of this Organization in 1923 for ten years, from 1924 to 1934. He was the secretary-treasurer of International Hahnemannian Association.

Dr. Roberts was one of the incorporators of the American Foundation for Homoeopathy. His distinguished services to this foundation as a Chairman of its Board of Trustees for a number of years were highly praised. Besides, for many years he was a member of the faculty of the post Graduate School under management of this foundation.

When the Homoeopathic Recorder was acquired by the International Hahnemannian Association in the year 1927, Dr. Roberts was selected to be its Editor-in-Chief until 1934.

Probably Dr. Roberts is the only and first man to serve in the U.S. Army Medical Corps during World War, with a rank of First Lieutenant.

He was master of homoeopathic philosophy and his command over homoeopathic materia medica was overwhelming. His "Study of Remedies by Comparison" is a classic work of materia media specially to the therapeutics of rheumatic fever. But his greatest work and contribution is "The Principles and Art of Cure by Homoeopathy" published in 1935. Dr. Roberts devoted his entire life to the interests and services of homoeopathy. His utmost aim was the prosperity and progress of homoeopathy. He was not only a very good teacher, author and philosopher, but also a very capable and remarkable prescriber and physician. Dr. Roberts was a very modest man. He was very humble and his life style was very simple. His no activity was aimed for personal gain. His aim and destination was welfare of homoeopathy. His long hours of research, writings, and teaching in the midst of a busy practice were his sacrifices to strengthen homoeopathy. He always attempted to make homoeopathic principles better understood and followed.

In every aspect of life Dr. Roberts stood as a strong and ardent supporter of homoeopathy.

DEMISE

On the 13th October 1950, this great philosopher and ideal follower of homoeopathy died in Brattleboro, Vermont.

HIS HOMOEOPATHIC WRITINGS

1. Study of Remedies by Comparison.
2. The Rheumatic Remedies.
3. Sensation as if.
4. The Principles and Art of Cure by Homoeopathy.

SOURCE MATERIAL

Homoeopathic Recorder, Volume LXVI.

Dr. Kulkarni Roy V. M.

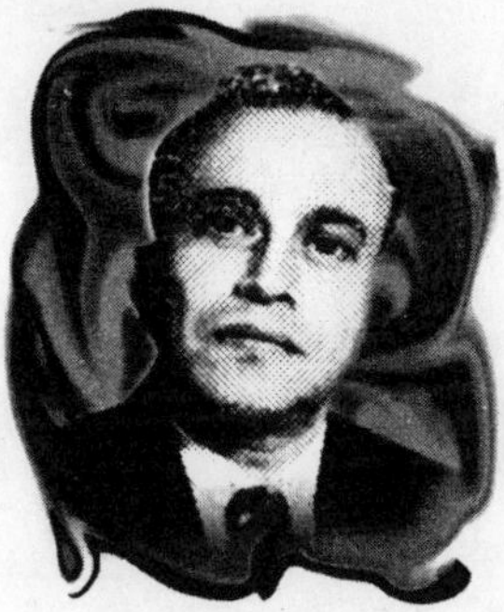

Born : 1908 Died : 07-11-1965

Dr. V.M. Kulkarni Roy was born in 1908 and died on November 7, 1965. In the field of homoeopathy his contribution has been great and most commendable as a physician, a pharmacist and a publisher. He was connected with the Bombay Homoeopathy Education Society and Bombay Homoeopathic Medical College.

Affirm joy in yourself . Don't wait passively for joy to come.

SECTION-S .... Page 219 to 256

S-1 ***Dr. Sahni, B.***
(Born: 17-01-1925 / Died: 26-10-1997) 220

S-2 ***Dr. Sankaran, P.***
(Born: 15-11-1922 / Died: 20-01-1979) 225

S-3 ***Dr. Sarkar, B.K.***
(Born: 27-12-1901 / Died: 06-02-1981) 228

S-4 ***Dr. Schmidt, Pierre***
(Born: 22-07-1894 / Died: 15-10-1987) 235

S-5 ***Dr. Schuessler, Whilhelm Heinrich***
(Born: 21-08-1821 / Died: 30-03-1898) 237

S-6 ***Dr. Sen, Suresh Chandra***
(Born: 01-08-1880 / Died: 26-03-1968)...............241

S-7 ***Dr. Sinha, G.N.*** (Died: 17-01-1959).....................242

S-8 ***Dr. Sircar, Mahendra Lal***
(Born: 02-11-1883 / Died: 24-02-1904) 243

Dr. B. Sahni

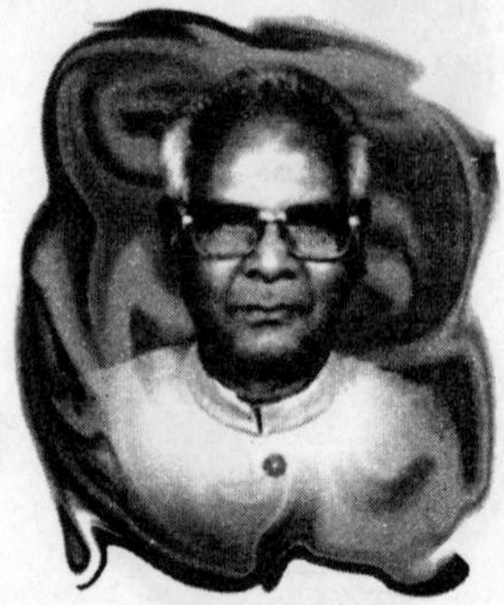

Born : 17-01-1925 Died : 26-10-1997

A PROFILE OF A DISCOVERER

Rare gift to the medical world in general and Homoeopathy in particular was made in the form of new discovery of Transmission of Homoeo Drug Energy Transmission from A Distance by great saint physician Dr. Bandhu Sahni.

Dr. Bandhu Sahni came from a very poor cultivator family. He was born on 17th January 1925 in a small village called Karkauli in the District of Darbhanga in Bihar. His early childhood is a tale of pain and penury. His father being a poor cultivator, found it difficult to maintain the family with his petty income. Dr. Sahni's extraordinary intelligence and zeal for acquiring knowledge at once attracted the notice of late Munsi Udit Narain of Rajnagar in Darbhanga, who is well know for his love for learning and magnamity. Under his loving care he lived with him and completed his matriculation in 1942. This made him realized that no sacrifice could be considered greater than one done for the sake of one's country. He left his studies and took active part in the freedom movement and was jailed on several occasions. It was during this period he was attracted towards Homoeopathy, which to him held promises of new awakening in the poor masses. It was a chanticleer of new dawn, which in turn would bring health and happiness to the suffering humanity.

Dr. Sahni, a man of indefatigable spirit and peerless character, again took up his studies and did his graduation from C.M. College Darbhanga. Afterwards he joined Basic Training School at Patna in 1948. Soon after finishing his BT course he was married to Dr. Sumitra Sahni, who too has done her basic training from the same school. Later both of them were appointed Assistant Teacher in Basic School at Kolhanta Patori in the district of Darbhanga, Bihar.

Section-S : Dr. Sahni, B.

At no stage of his career, though Dr. Sahni's interest in Homoeopathy reduced. Encouraged his interest made him complete his MD in Homoeopathy from Sathi Homoeopathic Medical College in Darbhanga. This encouraged him to establish a charitable Homoeopathic Dispensary under the Social Education Scheme. His wife has remained his constant companion in his entire endeavour ever since.

A voracious reader Dr. Sahni was always in quest to discover new phenomenon of nature. His love for learning always helped him climb fresh heights.

He kept his studies continued and while in service he did his post graduction twice. He did his MA first in Philosophy and then in Sociology. During the same time competed for service at Bhagalpur that Dr. Sahni came out with his discovery on Transmission of Homoeo Drug Energy. In recognition for his invaluable research many academic bodies and institutions for homoeopathic science has conferred upon him honorary degree and fellowship.

Dr. Sahni extended the philosophy of Dr. Hahnemann. His discovery of remote sensing technique of administering drugs, as against the conventional methods of administration of drugs through mouth in 1967, brought a revolutionary and far reaching changes in the field of medicine in general and Homoeopathy in particular. Today we can easily comprehend it in the light of distant transmission of various energy forms. In Dr. Sahnis scheme of things a single strand of hair is plucked from any part of the patients body which is then placed in the dynamic medicinal energy so that one end of the hair is submerged in the medicine, which in the liquid form, and other end remains free in the air to act as an antenna of a transmitter. Hair is used, as it is convenient to be taken from the patient. Any natural belonging of the patient can act as representative antenna for the patient. This antenna transmits the vital energy at a particular frequency specific to the patient. The vital energy signal traveling into the air are then received by the vital body of the patient acting as the receiver of a transmitter. Experiences over decades have proved that these vital energy signals can travel thousands of miles in no time without losing their intensity and effectiveness. In homoeopathy it is well understood that causation of all sickness lies within the person himself. As such a diseased person has a disoriented dynamic plane, which is needed to be resolved to normalcy. As such a dynamic medicine is needed. Dr. Hahnemann had earlier discovered the dynamic medicine by potentising the medicine by extracting out the energy level of it. As such all Homoeopathic medicines are not a commodities to be fed by mouth. They start acting as soon as they come in contact with the patient itself. Dr. Sahni added a new dimension to the mode of application of this dynamic medicine property by applying them from a distance by using the natural belonging of the patient. With varied experimentation on thousands of patients of various category it is now proved beyond doubt that dynamic medicine of Homoeopathy can be transmitted from a distance. Dr. Sahni's discovery is now a established system with thousands of followers all across the globe, so much so that he earned the lanurel of a physician, a messiah. In the forward of Dr. Sahni's book "Transmission of Homoeo Drug Energy From A Distance" Dr. Jugal Kishore, former President of Central Council of Homoeopathy rates him even higher than the father of Homoeopathy, Dr. Hahnemann. He writes "Apparently the author (Dr. B. Sahni) has traveled much beyond Hahnemann when the latter advocated transmission of drug energy by olfaction". Dr. Sahni's method of application of medicine is now recognized by his followers as Sahni effect. A new concept to health has been added with his discovery. In order to bring into application his remote sensing technique and furtherance of the scope of drug transmission and its scientific parameters, Dr. B. Sahni laid the foundation of Research Institute of Sahni Drug Transmission & Homoeopathy in 1970, which was later on registered under the Society Registration Act, 1860. With the initial activity of propagation, research and training through non-formal basis, the institute is now marching ahead with healthcare through drug transmission by its various free clinics spread over the country.

In 1974, Dr. B. Sahni travelled extensively to share his valuable experiences as a result of which his students are now distributed worldwide. His efforts has brought tremendous response from the masses and the intellectuals alike and proved the efficacy of his principle and methods of treatment beyond doubts. With his excellence in the art of application of medicine especially the subject of philosophy, medicine and reportorial analysis and vast experiences accumulated in them attached many disciple who used to come to him from every corner of the world. Now his message has spread worldwide. Dr. B. Sahni besides being a discoverer was a great soul with caring hearts, which won over the thousands of his followers. He was elected President of the

Section-S : Dr. Sahni, B.

Homoeopathic Medical Association of India, Bihar State Branch for two terms. Later on he was elevated to the National post of Vice President of The Homoeopathic Medical Association of India. His sincerity and caliber in Homoeopathy attracted Government of Bihar who was pleased to nominate him as the member of the Bihar State Homoeopathic Board. He served the Board with his intelligence to develop it to the extent of making academic nature of Homoeopathy more effective system of Medicine. A well learned Dr. Sahni was invited on many occasion at various seminars to present his paper. In 1977 he presented his paper at International Homoeopathic Congress, Vigyan Bhawan, New Delhi. This was introduction of his subject of Drug Transmission to the Homoeopathic fraternity of the world. Learned delegates from all over the world listened to the discoverer and he was appreciated widely for his new exploration in the field of medicine. Later on he was also invited to present his paper by the Indian Science Congress on three occasions. Chairman of the scientific session were impressed with his presentation and delivered remarks in appreciation. His paper was also presented at International Homoeopathic Congress at Calcutta in 1989 and in many of the national and regional seminars.

Dr. Sahni served medical institutions in varied capacity. He was visiting Professor to the B.H. Medical College and Hospital at Patna. He was made Vice Chairman of the Institute of Healing & Alternative Therapy at Patna. He also served National Editorial Board of History of Indian Homoeopathy.

Dr. Shani's love for books was well known. His vast collection of books on the subject of medicine alone has now become a treasure house of knowledge in the form of a library at *The Research Institute of Sahni Drug Transmission & Homoeopathy.* His collection of rare books is still stored in this library.

A renowned author of Transmission of Homoeo Drug Energy From A Distance, a book which is now published in 4 editions opens a vast field of research in energy medicines. He also authored many other books and his articles were published in various journals of Homoeopathy. His interest in propagating initiated in him to write at regular intervals as such he took up journalism and founded publication of two journal - one in Hindi and other in English. He was founder editor of quarterly Homoeopathic Journal Homoeo Tarang in Hindi and The Journal of Homoeo Transmission in English. Dr. Sahni became a legend in the field of medicine and is remembered in various story of cure related to him. His interest in healing the sufferings of ailing patient was widely appreciated. A man with heart full of passion for helping to relieve the suffering can be well imagined as patient from all over the country used to come to him for their treatments. He offered his services to many of the Medical centers and has the distinction of organizing many medical camps to bring his discovery available to the needy poor patient in remote villages. He traveled from village to village to help the poor. Still today he is remembered for his services.

Dr. Sahni's thirst for helping and propagating the truth of art of healing encouraged him to travel abroad. He went to Switzerland, Germany, France, England, Belgium, USA and other country, where he was welcomed as scientist. He also taught many students during his stay at various countries. At San Francisco he worked with a AIDS patient and tried to discover the cure for it. He helped in the establishment of Healing Centre of San Francisco. His health gradually started succumbing to the pressure of work and was paralyzed after a cerebral stroke to bed in 1990 being helped with his own discovery he lived on bed for more than seven years. Still lying on his sick bed he used to deliver lessons on his subject to the entire disciples who used to come to seek consultation for their difficulties. He started a weekly study programme being managed from his bedside. His every moment of life was not lived in vain.

Recognizing his services to the Homoeopathy and his discovery Dr. Sahni was felicitated posthumously by the Central Council of Homoeopathy, a Govt. of India statutory body, during its silver jubilee celebration in 1999. Vice President of India Dr. S.D. Sharma presented the memento to Dr. B. Sahni, which was received by his son Dr. M.K. Sahani. A grateful Council paid its homage to this saint by honoring and recognizing his services. Variously described as a healer saint, a messiah and a scientist healer Dr. B. Sahni, a down to the earth person shall remain alive in the hearts of millions.

Much before he left for his heavenly abode on 26th October 1997, Dr. B. Sahni enjoyed the great task of ameliorating the pains of humanity through his remote sensing technique of distant application of medicine.

Section-S : Dr. Sahni, B.

Dr. P. Sankaran

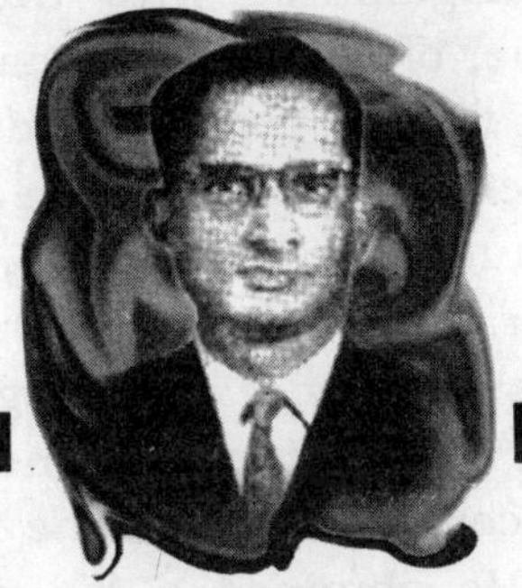

Born : 15-11-1922

Died : 20-01-1979

Dr. P. Sankaran was born on the 15th November 1922 in Madras, India. His father shifted to Bombay when he was 3 to 4 years old. He began his schooling here, but before the could complete it, his father died, leaving the family in a poor financial condition. The family of ten siblings was separated and were sent to various places to be supported by relatives. He went to Madras to say with his paternal uncle Dr. Sharma, an Ayurvedic practitioner. Here he was put in a college where both Ayurveda and Allopathy were taught, and qualified with a Licenciate in India Medicine (LIM). After working in a few jobs, he somehow managed to start his own practice in he early 1950's, and was practising allopathy predominantly. Within 2-3 years of starting his practice, he fell sick and was not relieved by the best allopathic treatment of the day, but was cured of his ailment by a homoeopath (described in "My Conversion to Homoeopathy"). This removed his scepticism and the became an ardent learner. In 1955-56, he got the opportunity to got to London, where he studied in the Royal London Homoeopathic Hospital under famous teachers like Sir John Weir, Margery M. Blackie, alva Benjamin, Foubister and other. It must be mentioned that the dominant emphasis in the Royal Hospital was on the Kentian method, with emphasis on the repertory and mind symptoms, etc. During this time, he also met Elizabeth Wright Hubbard, who invited him to New York. He came back to Bombay and restarted his practice with added vigour. As this practice grew in the Bombay suburb of Santa Cruz, he also started teaching in the Homoeopathic College and became Honorary Physician at the Govt. Homoeopathic Hospital. He married in 1959 and had a son in 1960.

Section-S : Dr. Sankaran, P.

He founded and edited the Journal of Homoeopathic Medicine, which was later amalgamated into the Indian Journal of Homoeopathic Medicine, of which he remained the editor till the end. In 1965, he went to New York to study under Dr. E. Wright Hubbard. She was much impressed by him and asked him to be a teacher (instead of a student) in the course. After hearing his first lecture on Lachesis, Dr. Hubbard wrote, "Dr. Sankaran's talk was so captivating with his knowledge of zoology, botany, psychology and homoeopathy, and with such a fine sense of humour that "The Sankarans" would be competition for "The Beatles", if only there were four of them!" He obtained a diploma in Homoeopathic Therapeutics from there.

In India, he was one of the main persons responsible for the propagation of the Repertory. At that time, the dominant school of practice was that of the Calcutta Homoeopaths, with an emphasis on the Materia Medica to the near exclusion of the repertory. One of the first works he authored was the Card Repertory, which was a refinement of Boger's Card Repertory. Not finding a publisher, he started his own Publishing Company, and later on went on to write and publish 36 small booklets. He was one of the leading figures in the profession and was responsible for the organisation of many meetings, symposia and conferences which were purely scientific and non-political. Here he was much supported by his close friends who included Dr. J.N. Kanjilal (Calcutta), Dr. S.P. Koppikar (Madras), Dr. Sarabhai Kapadia (Bombay) and Dr. Jugal Kishore (Delhi). He was closely associated with Dr. L.D. Dhawale and Dr. S.R. Phatak, both great admirers of Boger. He was a member of the first Central Council of Homoeopathy which was instrumental in formulating standards and guidelines for homoeopathic colleges. He was one of the instructors in the Teachers' Orientation course where he taught the repertory to teachers of Homoeopathic colleges. He presented papers in various international conferences. He was known for his warmth, his sense of humour, skill in communication, diplomacy, sincerity and a remarkable open-mindedness. He investigated diverse areas of science trying to improve and advance Homoeopathy. He worked on Kirlian Photography, Bowel Nosodes, Boyd's Emmanometer, did provings, experimented with the repetition of remedies etc. Besides Homoeopathy, he was interested in such varied things as Travelling, Psychology, Photography, and was learning the musical instrument, Veena.

Section-S : Dr. Sankaran, P.

He practised in two places in Bombay, visiting each on alternate days. His practice was extremely busy, and he kept up his hectic schedule of practice, teaching, editing, organising etc., till the very end. His health gave way. In 1978, cancer in the second stage was diagnosed. He lived for 6 months after the diagnosis during which time, in between his pains, he managed to complete three of his booklets and write the last one, "The Selection of the Similimum and Management of the Patient."

Dr. P. Sankaran passed away on 20th January 1979 in Bombay.

Dr. B.K. Sarkar

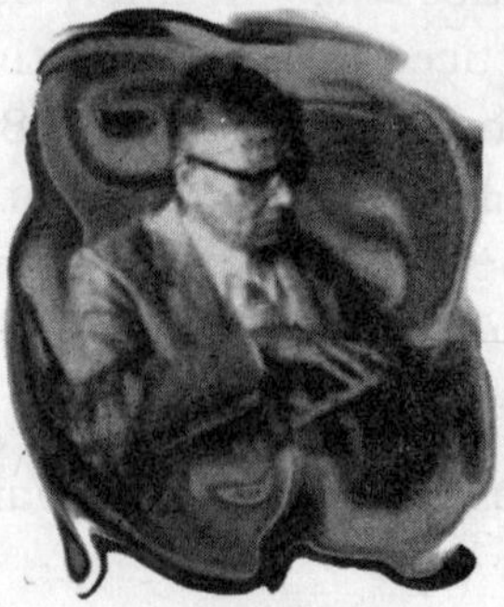

Born : 27-12-1901 **Died : 06-02-1981**

If the age-old theories of the invisible mechanisms and unseen hands of the providence or destiny has any truth in them, history is full of such men and women who started with different goals and ended up with some very different achievements, and in few exceptional instances they suffered in consequences personal hardships and privations but the path, the ideology which they cherished and served flourished. The science and the ideologies gained, the man suffered. Homoeopathy has its own share of a small band of persons who left their well-cushioned life, livelihood and opulence and came to serve homoeopathy, a revolution in the world of medicine and suffered in consequence. They lost what they had, homoeopathy acquired, what it did not have the list of such revolutionaries like Hahnemann, Hull, Mahendra Lal Sircar, and B.K. Sarkar is not very long but very unique, very glorious, very inspiring and very, very memorable. Dr. B.K. Sarkar left his career, job, opulence and well-earned luxuries to promote and propagate the cause of homoeopathy. While he acquired a new indentity, a new image, a new fame of a warrior, his family suffered economically in home and socially in the eyes of his less gifted and more earning colleagues. Dr. Sarkar made homoeopathy richer and his family poorer.

ANCESTORS & FAMILY

Dr. Sarkar belonged a well-to-do family. His maternal grandfather was an allopathic physician in the employment of B.N. Railway. All of his 5 brothers were educated and well-placed in life.

BIRTH

He was the second son of his parents and was born on Friday,

Section-S : Dr. Sarkar, B.K.

the 27th December, 1901 at Chairmar Sahi in Midnapur town in West Bengal.

MEDICAL EDUCATION

He did his Graduation in Medicine from Calcutta University in the year 1925. After completing his M.D. he became house physician in the Carmichael Medical Collage (Presently R.G. Kar Medical College and Hospital). He worked on the same post from 1925 to 1927. Dr. Sarkar secured first position in the M.D. examination and he was honoured with Gold Medal and Honours in Physiology and Medicine. Throughout his whole academic career he secured scores of scholarship and prizes, among which Aghore Prakash Scholarship, Rakhal Ghosh Prize, Guptu Scholarship deserve special mention. He received Silver Medal in Physics and Botany for standing first in both the subjects.

MEDICAL PRACTICE & CONVERSION TO HOMOEOPATHY

In the year 1928 he started his private allopathic practice in Calcutta and subsequently joined Merchant Navy as a Physician/ Surgeon on Ship.

His very close friend and equally talented classmate Dr. Sanat Kumar Ghosh's father was a renowned homoeopathic physician of North Calcutta. Although Dr. Sarkar and Dr. Sanat Ghosh could not agree easily to what Senior Dr. Ghosh said about homoeopathy but they could hardly overlook the cures and relief that he gave to his patients.

He started reading homoeopathic books and literatures during the long lonely voyages to sea. In the year 1935 he started practicing homoeopathy on Mohini Mohan Road, at Bhowanipur. Very soon his sincerity and knowledge in homoeopathy was recognised and he was accepted as a learned and well-informed homoeopath in West Bengal, and then in India.

In 1952 he appeared at the D.M.S. examination like any ordinary student and received not only Honours in Organon but the first Gold Medal of the D.M.S. examination.

CONTRIBUTIONS TO HOMOEOPATHY

Educational

1. In 1936 he became Professor of Homoeopathic Materia Medica and Organon and a visiting physician in the

outdoor of Bengal Allen Homoeopathic Medical College and Hospital.

2. In 1948 he became the Principal of D.N. De Homoeopathic Medical College, Calcutta.
3. From 1944 to 1960 he became the Principal and Trustee Member of Midnapur Homoeopathic Medical College.
4. Nominated as a member of the General Council and State Faculty of Homoeo pathic Medicine, West Bengal, since its inception from 1942.
5. Elected as Chairman of the Executive Committee of the Homoeopathic State Faculty for 3 terms from 1950 to 1960.

Organisational

1. Chairman of the Reception Committee, Registered Homoeopathic Practititoner's Conference, West Bengal in the year 1945.
2. President, Bihar Homoeopathic Science Congress, 1953.
3. President, All India Institute of Homoeopathy, 1953.
4. President, Third Session of All India Homoeopathic Congress, New Delhi, 1953.
5. President, Second All India Homoeopathic Conference, Madras, 1962.

Legislative

1. Chairman: The Homoeopathic Pharmacopoeia Committee, Government of India.
2. Member: Research and Technical Sub-committee of Homoeopathic Advisory Committee, Government of India.
3. Member: Homoeopathic Advisory Committee, Government of India.
4. Member: Homoeopathic Education Sub-committee, Government of India.
5. Member: Homoeopathic Sub-committee of the Drugs Technical Advisory Committee, Government of India.

Research

1. Chief Controller: Homoeopathic Drug Research Committee, Midnapur Homoeopathic College unit.

Section-S : Dr. Sarkar, B.K.

Professional

1. Honorary Visiting Physician : Marwari Relief Calcutta.
2. Visiting Physician : D.N. De Homoeopathic College & Hospital, Midnapur Homoeopathic Medical College and Hospital.

Literary

1. *Journalism :*

Editor :

- Hahnemannian Gleanings.
- Hahnemann Bangla.
- Homoeopathic Herald.
- Homoeopathic Chikitsak.

In these journals he published hundreds of articles, reviews of publications, comments on legislations and activities.

2. *Original Books :*

- A Commentary on Organon of Medicine. This is a textbook of many Boards and Councils for Homoeopathy.
- Essentials of Homoeopathic Philosophy.
- Homoeopathic Prasanga (Bangla).
- Drug Relationship.
- Upto Date with Nosodes.

3. *Other Writings :*

Historical :

- Hahnemann, the Rebel and the Reformer.
- History of Medicine with Special Reference to Homoeopathy.
- A Historical and Critical Study of the Evolution of Medical Philosophy in the West.
- History of the Introduction and Spread of Homoeopathy in India.
- Dr. Mahendra Lal Sircar — In Memoriam.

Homoeopathy and Philosophy :

- The Truth in Homoeopathy.
- The Totality of Symptoms — Its Philosophical Significance.

- The Totality of Symptoms — The Art.
- Different Grades of Truth and Reality.
- Mechanism, Organism and Life.
- Holism and Homoeopathy.
- The Causality of the Whole and the Field of Organism.
- Notes on Living Organisms, Matter and Mind.
- Causal Medicine and Homoeopathy.
- The Notio of Causality in Relation to Organism.
- The Body-Life-Mind Puzzle.
- Individuality and Personality.
- Metaphysical Discussion about Illness, Its Causes and Cure.

Homoeopathy and Science:

- The Development of Scientific Spirit : The Special Prerogative of Modern Age.
- Science and Matter.
- The Nature of Scientific Methodology Relevant for the Study of Man and Medicine in General and Homoeopathy in Particular.
- Homoeopathy in the Light of Modern Physical Science.
- Science and Scientific Truth.
- Methods of Science and Their Applications to Homoeopathy.
- Homeopathy and Modern Scientific System of Medicine.
- Homoeopathy and the Science of Medicine.
- Relationship between Medicine and Biology.
- The Difficulties in the Study of Human Biology.
- Scientificity of Homoeopathy.

Homoeopathy and Modern Medicine:

- Ideological Conflict between Homoeopathy and the Modern Scientific Medicine.
- Illusions of Modern Scientific Medicine in Connection with Statistics and Prophylactic Measures against Infectious Diseases.
- The Place of Homoeopathy in Preventive Medicine.
- The Relation of Homoeopathic Materia Medica to Physiology and Pathology.

Section-S : Dr. Sarkar, B.K.

- Allergy and Homoeopathy.
- Anaphylaxis, Immunity and Homoeopathy.
- Mechanism of Production of Physical symptoms in Illness.
- The Modern Conception of Psycho-somatic Medicine and Homoeopathy.
- Fundamental Differences between Orthodox Medicine and Homoeopathy.
- Conception of Infection - Modern and Hahnemannian Medical Diagnosis.
- Disease in the Eye of a Physician.
- Fundamental Medical Ideas of Hahnemann in the Light of Modern Medicine.
- The Root Problem of Medicine.
- Fundamental Ideas Regarding Medicine in General and Homoeopathy in Particular.
- Psycho-somatic Medicine and Homoeopathy.
- Separate Point Statistics and Homoeopathy.
- The Study of Homeopathic Drugs from the Standpoint of Endocrinology.
- Homoeopathy, both a Science and an Art.
- The place of Disease Diagnosis in the Homoeopathic System of Medicine.
- Modern Conception of Tuberculosis and its Comparative Study from Homoeo-pathic Point of View.
- Homoeopathy in Treatment of Diseases of Modern Age due to Nervous Strain.

On Hahnemann :

- Hahnemann (In Memoriam).
- Hahnemann, the Bacteriologist.
- Hahnemann — Birth-Centenary Oration.
- Homoeopathy, a Saving Grace for the Suffering Humanity.
- The Story of Publication of the Sixth Edition of Hahnemann's Organon.
- Introspection.
- An Anecdote.

Homoeopathic Polemics :

- Editorial Articles of the Journal of the Indian Medical Association, July 1949: Homoeopathy.
- Homoeopathy Vindicated — A Rejoinder.
- Hahnemann's Prevision of Bacteriology— A Misconception by Dr. G. Dirghangi.
- A Comment on 'Hahnemann's Prevision of Bacteriology — A Misconception'.
- Is It Correct for a Homoeopath to Say that Hahnemann was the Father of Bacteriology? By Shri Bhagwan Das.
- A Comment: Condemnation of Homoeopathy and its Refutal.
- Hahnemann's Doctrine of Psora and the Homoeopathic Treatment of Skin Diseases, by J. Paterson.
- A Criticism of Dr. Paterson's Exposition of Hahnemann's Doctrine of Psora.
- Is Homoeopathy a Complete System of Medicine?
- The Definition of a Homoeopathic Physican.
- Why the Homoeopathic Therapeutical Law, though Strictly Scientific, Does Not Meet with General Acceptance?
- Dogmatism Dies Hard.
- Is Homoeopathy Progressive?
- A Gap in Homoeopathy.
- The Need of Aggressive Homoeopathy.
- Homoeopathy Pure and Mixed.
- Vision of an Ideal Physician.
- The Same Old Story.
- Homoeopathy.
- Modern Scientific Medicine.
- Similia Similibus Curentur.

Section-S : Dr. Sarkar, B.K.

Dr. Pierre Schmidt

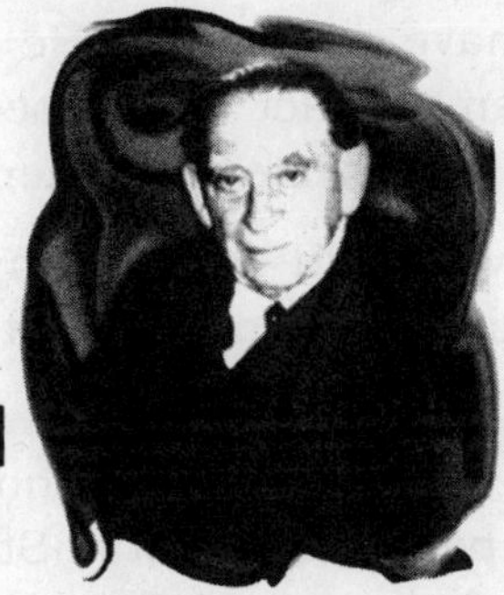

Born : 22-07-1894 **Died : 15-10-1987**

Pierre Schmidt, M.D., was born on the 22nd of July, 1894. He received his early education in Geneva. Schmidt came to know about homoeopathy in 1918, in London, where he saw the results of homoeopathic treatment during an epidemic of flu. Schmidt met both Dr. J.H. Clarke and Dr. John Weir while he was in London.

In 1922 he went to United States and learned homoeopathy from Austin and Gladwin. At that time both, Austin and Gladwin, were working as the core faculty at the first session of the American Foundation School. Schmidt returned to Geneva and set up his practice there. He taught pure homoeopathy to several generations of physicians in Europe.

He wrote many pamphlets and helped in editing the final General Repertory of Kent. He translated the Organon into French. Dr. Gladwin always referred to Schmidt as *Sunshine*.

Robert Schore, M.D., Dr. Jost Kunzli's student, paid a brief visit to Dr. Schmidt in 1979. He recalls this visit:

"I was impressed with the grandeur of his office, a very large room containing hundreds of volumes of homoeopathic texts and journals, many carefully bound in leather. His custom built wood remedy cabinets were magnificent. His examination room was a smaller adjacent room containing an exam table, an instrument table, and an acupuncture chart on the wall. I browsed around while I waited about twenty minutes for him to enter the room. I will always remembers the first thing he said to me (in a very abrupt manner): 'What questions do you have?' I had gone there just to meet him and chat about homoeopathy in Europe, and I found myself intimated as if I was in an audience with the Pope! I introduced myself as a student of his student, Dr. Jost Kunzli, who arranged for me to meet him. We had a very brief conversation. He said that it was very important to study everything about homoeopathy and to have questions. He also mentioned that acupuncture could be an adjunct to homoeopathy as long as the doctor was familiar with both systems of therapy."

In 1925, he was involved in establishing the Liga Medicorum Homoeopathic Internationalis, an international organization of classical homoeopathic physicians.

Schmidt had a 3000+ volume library of homoeopathic literature, which is now in the occupancy of a trust in St. Gallien, Switzerland. This library is now used for research purposes.

Dr. Whilhelm Heinrich Schuessler

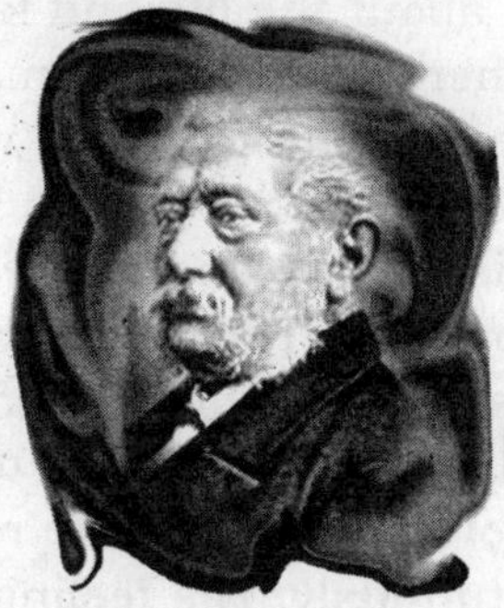

Born : 21-08-1821 Died : 30-03-1898

BIRTH

Germany has remained a land of small population and great ideas; the land of original thinkers and revolutionary reformers; the land of discoverers or discoveries and investions and inventors; the land of Bismarck and Kaiser and Hitler and Rommel, the land of Dante and Goethe and Bothoven and Max Mueller: the land of Marx and Schosenhulr and Freud and Einstein, Germany is the land of Hahnemann and Schuessler.

Wilhelm Heinrich Schuessler was born in Germany. The place was Zwischenalm in the Grand Duchy of Oldenburg. The day was 21st of August in 1821.

EDUCATION

His youth and early manhood were spent in acquiring an extensive knowledge in vairous branches of human knowledge. At an early age, he perfected his knowledge of Philology for which he was endowed with rare talent. He knew Latin, Greek, French, Italian, Spanish and English. He used to study Sanskrit too. He was a much sought after private tutor of languages. Thus, he prepared the basis for his latter studies in the Universities. Only at a mature age and a much later date Schuessler could carry out his long desired wish of entering a university. He studied in the universities of Papers, Berlin and Giessen where he studied for five terms. He studied further for three terms in Prague and obtained his M.D. On August 14, 1857, he received the license required in those days for settling as a physician. He settled as a Homoeopathic Physician in Oldenburg.

FAMILY

But little is known about the life and family of the creator and founder of Biochemic Therapy. He was unmarried. He had very few, nearly none, of his near relatives living when he shot to fame. Nothing touching was found in the papers he left behind him. The repeated requests of his friends and followers could not persuade him to write his autobiography. He was convinced of the importance and scientific exactness of the therapy created by him. He was reticent and modest in every thing which touched him personally. His fees during whole of his medical life remained low and many families he treated gratuitously. His feeling for the not so-affluent fellow beings are amply shown in his last will and testament. He was a man of science and possessed a singular straight-forwardness, which sometimes, especially when something was imputed to him who he could not reconcile with his views, passed over into roughness and he never cared whether his opponents were men of destination or common people. Free from the fear of men, he went his way without looking whether he gave offence on the right hand or on the left; and full of conviction of his principles, he defended his cause against all.

Through his system of tissue therapy Schuessler became known throughout the civilized world and patients from all parts of the world come to him. But success could not infuse pride or arrogance in him. He remained the plain and simple man he had been from his youth. He lived alone in a large mansion, a life of an educated peasant, regular and humble, and his personal requirements were very limited. Until the end of his life, his attention and attempts were directed to the cure of his patients and the development of the system of medicine, which he has given birth to.

In 1832, Johnm Ernst Stapf, a renowned friend and disciple of Hahnemann, the founder of Homoeopathy, wrote in the first homoeopathic journal of the world "Archiv fuer die Homoeopathische Heikunst." "All the essential component parts of the human body are great remedies." Again, in the same periodical, we find "All the constituents of the human body act in such organs principally when they have a function." Schuessler himself, in his first article admitted that his theory owed its origin to the inspiration from the few phrases of an article entitled. "Circle of Life", (Kreislanf des Lebens) by Professor Moleschott of Rome, in which he had said, "The Structure and function of the organs depend upon the presence of the necessary balanced quantities of the inorganic constituents."

Section-S : Dr. Schuessler, W.H.

In March, 1973, Schuessler published an article in German entitled *"Abegkurja The Pic"* which has been translated in English as "Abridged Therapeutics" in which he said, "About a years ago I intend to find out by experiments on the sick if it were not possible to heal them, provided their diseases were curable at all with some substances that are natural, i.e. physiological functional remedies." Five months after the article was published Dr. Lorbacher, of Leipsig, came out with some criticism in the same Journal. Boerieke & Dewey claim the name of the article to be "An Abridged Homoeopathic Therapeutics." While E.L. Peery in his "General Sketch of the Biochemic System of Medicine" and Dr. J. B. Chapman in his "Dr Schuessler's Biochemisty" name it as "Shortened Therapeutics" and as "Abridged Therapy" respectively. However, T.L. Bradford, the immortal historian of homoeopathy in his 'Homoeopathic Bibliogrpahy of the U.S.A. - 1825 to 1891' lists the title as 'Abridged Therapeutics; founded upon Histology and Cellular Pathology, with an appendix giving special directions for the application of the inorganic cell step and indications of the underlying conditions of morbid states of tissues and it was the authorised translation by M. Doccti Walter in 1880. Dr. Schuessler's reply to the criticism ran through seven issue of the journal giving details of the new system of treatment. Dr. H.C. Luyties of St. Louis MO rendered the English translation of the article.

In 1874, M/s Boericke & Tafel of U.S.A. published a booklet of 44 pages titled as : 'The Twelve Tissue Remedies and their use in trituration of Dr. Schuessler, recommended for investigation by Dr. C. Hering". The original work of Dr. Schuessler went through 25 editions with additions and extensions by the author during his lifetime.

DEMISE

The wish of his many adherents of home and around the world that the founder and the honoured master of Biochemic system of treatment might be permitted to labor for a few more years in advancing the work of his life was not fulfilled. He has reached the age of 77 years. Upto March 14th, he was in good health and then suddenly he suffered a stroke but he recovered very soon and he was able to finish on the afternoon of the next days, i.e. 15th of March the last proof of the last sheet of the 25th edition of his 'Abridged Therapy'. This was fated to be his last work. Soon his condition was seriously grave and he remained unconscious for several days. And the boy who excelled in Philology, a homoeopath who distinguished himself as a physician, a discoverer, who found a new system of healing died in the evening on 30th of March 1898. The morning of life was spent in accumulation of knowledge, the day in healing the sick, the noon in the thoughts, discovery and establishment of his own system of healing, the evening ended early to mingle with the darkness of night, the darkness of death. And in the evening of his life, the life left the body, the body, which was his object of study, Biochemical analysis and Biochemical treatment. The greatman was carried in a mourning procession of his disciples and followers, friends and patients to the grave on tuesday, the 5th of April on a Sunny Spring morning.

The atoms that had been conjoined together in this great son of the earth not merely for joy and grief but for the fulfilment of higher duties were restored to the mother earth. Very soon, elements on the body were to mix with the elements of the earth around but the traces of his earthly life, his foot prints on the history of human knowledge, his marks in world of medicine will remain forever, and ever, and ever. Shakespear said in Hamlet,

"He was a man, take him for all in all,
I shall not look upon his like again."

Schuessler's therapy has been used by laymen practitioners, allopaths, homoeopaths and biochemic practitioners. Millions of human beings have been treated and cured by the system. Who have derived benefit from its healing powers it has been a pain killer, a health given and a life saver. Schuessler's contribution for them has been relief, health and new life.

Schuessler gave a new direction to the medical thinking. The modern medical science recognizes the deficiency diseases due to insufficient intake or assimilation of it and realizes the necessity to makeup for the deficiency in vitamins, hormones and enzymes, minerals, etc. Schuessler can be rightly acclaimed as the father of Deficiency Therapy.

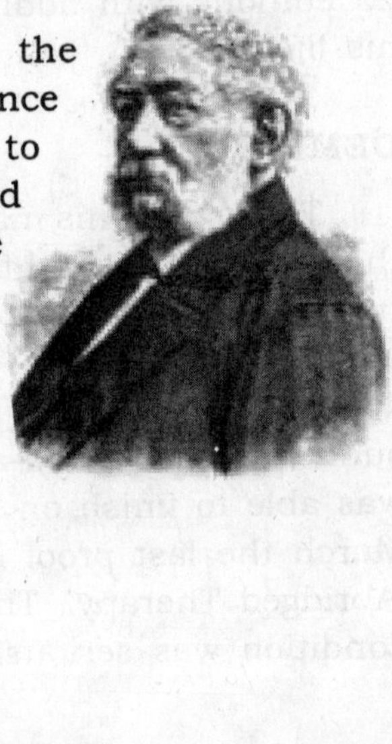

Dr. Suresh Chandra Sen

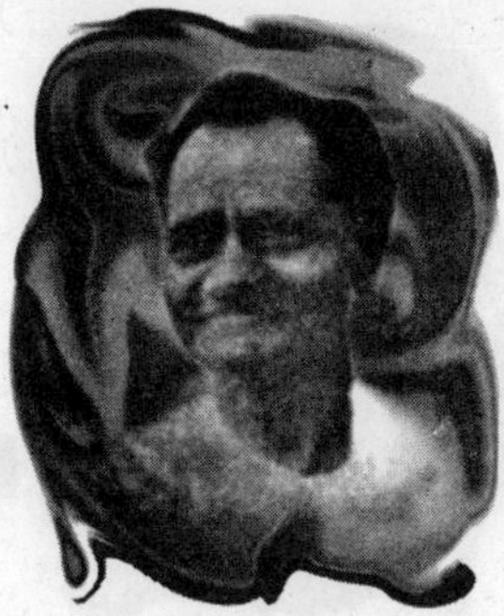

Born : 01-08-1880 Died : 26-03-1968

Late Rev. Dr. Suresh Chandra Sen, M.D. was a man of philanthropic deads, and indefatigable energy. He was born on August 1, 1880 in Dacca District of earstwhile Bengal.

The Government Homoeopathic Sanatorium, Nowgaon, Madhya Pradesh, owns its growth to his philanthropic efforts.

His achievements are the establishment of Homoeopathic Sanatorium, appointment of homoeopathic doctors in State Medical Services, creation of a post of Asstt. Surgeon for Homoeopathy is Class II Gazetted cadre, a status at par with allopathy in Madhya Pradesh Medical Services, decision of the State Govt. for establishment of a State Degree College of Homoeopathy, establishment of the Board of Homoeopathic and Biochemic Systems of Medicine in M.P. in 1951, and publication of Journal of M.P. Homoeopathic Board. He went to America in 1906. When homoeopathic system of treatment was there at its peak, he took to study of homoeopathy and graduated from Philadalphia. After returning to India, Dr. Sen started his practice at Calcutta. Later he practiced at Raipur, Bilaspur and lastly at Jabalpur where he reached his acme of life.

He was the second President of the M.P. Homeopathic Board after the demise of Dr. K. L. Daftari in 1955, and after the reorganization of the states, he was the Chairman of the Mahakoshal Board of Homoeopathic Medicines. In 1959 when the State Govt. reconstituted the Board after the reorganization, he was nominated as the President of the Board, the office which he held till 1962. The passing away of Dr. S.C. Sen on March 26, 1968 is an irreparable loss. In him we lost a great philosopher, pioneer, creator and a guide.

Dr. G.N. Sinha

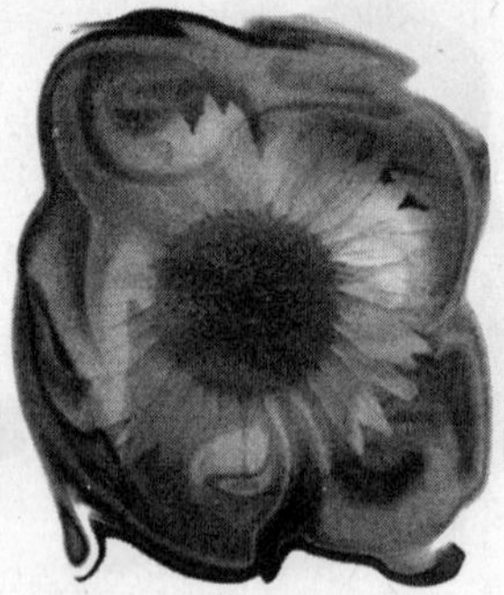

Died : 17-01-1959

Dr. G.N. Sinha, M.D., was a great homoeopath and a great teacher. He worked both as a Registrar and then for many years as the Principal of the Calcutta Homoeopathic Medical College. He expired on January 17, 1959.

Dr. Mahendra Lal Sircar

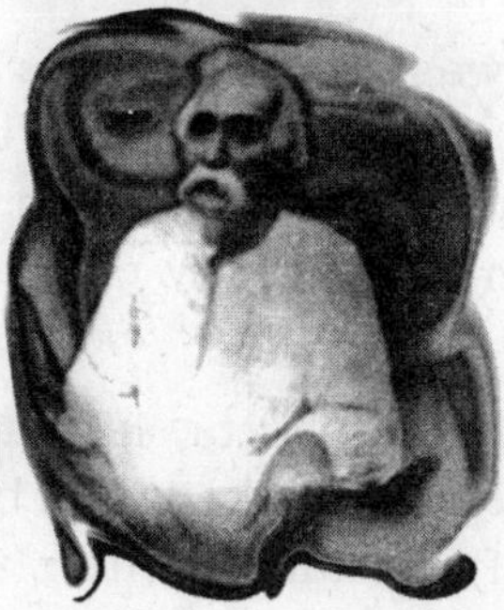

Born : 02-11-1883 **Died : 24-02-1904**

"That sanctity which settles on the memory of a great man, ought, upon a double motive to be vigilantly sustained by his countrymen; first, out of gratitude to him as one column of the national grandeur; secondly with a practical purpose of transmitting unimpaired to posterity the benefit of ennobling models."

To the benefit of this principle none amongst the great men of modern India is better entitled than the subject of this brief sketch, whether regarded as a physician, a patriot, or as a man, who had made considerable personal sacrifice for truth and his country. Few among the noteworthy personages of our country would more assiduously shrink from the public gaze, or shun with a more sensitive persistency the "fierce light" which, in this prying age, beats upon the inner lives of eminent men. But a man of his transcendent merit, as a successful practitioner of the healing art, as an erudite scholar, as an eminent scientist, fired with zeal for the regeneration of his country through the agency of science must necessarily be before the public, and that public was, in his case, almost world-wide. He was known not only throughout India, but his fame spread to Europe and America. His advice was asked even from Australia.

Dr. Sircar was born of exceedingly poor parents in an obscure village of the name of Paikpara, in the District of Howrah, in Bengal, on the 2nd of November 1833. He comes of the stock from which have sprung the actual tillers of the soil in this country, but certainly not from what are called the lower orders of society. He comes of the Vaisya caste. Dr. Sircar was not at all ashamed of the fact that he came into the world, unheralded by any reputation whatever on the part of his ancestors. For are not the world's greatest men, the pioneers of thought and culture, their own ancestors? He took the highest pride in this, that he was born of parents who had "passed into the skies."

At the age of 5 he was brought by his mother with an infant brother of 6 months to the house of her brothers, Babus Iswar Chandra Ghosh and Mahesh Chandra Ghosh, in Calcutta (Nebutola). He was never away from that locality endeared as it was by early associations.

Shortly after arrival at Calcutta, his father died at Paikpara, when only 32 years old. He had to be taken back to Paikpara on the occasion of the *sradh* of this father. After a short stay there, his mother, now a widow, brought back her sons to her brothers' where they remained for good.

His mother survived her husband's death for about 4 years, and died of cholera when she was about 32 years of age. It is remarkable that Mahendra Lal, the first born of his parents, was born when his mother was 24 years of age, a rather unusual age for a Hindu female to bear her first child.

The rudiments of his vernacular education was obtained in a neighbouring *patshala* under a *Gurumahasay,* and shortly after, the rudiments of his English education under the late Babu Thakur Das Dey, to whom he remained attached to the last.

At the age of seven he was put in the school of David Hare. Shortly after his admission Hare died. On the burial of this philanthropist under remarkable circumstances, Dr. Sircar held a distinct recollection.

In 1850, Dr. Sircar obtained a junior scholarship which enabled him to pass from the Hare School to the Hindu (afterwards the Presidency) College, where he soon distinguished himself as one of its brightest gems. It was while at this noted seminary of learning that he laid in a varied stock of knowledge — literary, philosophical, historical, scientific.

While as yet at school, science had already marked him for her own. He used to read Milner's *Tour through Creation,* a popular scientific work, with an avidity which was remarkable for a lad of his tender years. In a speech delivered at the time of laying the foundation-stone of the Science-Association, on March 27, 1890, by his Excellency Lord Lansdowne, Dr. Sircar referred to the incident which gave an impetus to his dominating scientific bias, with a rare tact and delicacy which is peculiarly his own, thus:

"My Lord, I knew a lad of 14 to 15, when I was of the same age myself, a lad not at all remarkable for intelligence, but who had what is called some thirst for knowledge, and a little enthusiasm in the pursuit of knowledge, who would feel an unspeakable pleasure in the possession of knowledge......... I remember an anecdote of this lad, my Lord..... With the characteristics of mind, just mentioned, he was naturally fond of reading scientific books. One day while reading Milner's *Tour through Creation* he came across the discovery of Sir William Herschell that the sun was not a fixed body in space, but with his planets and their satellites, was in motion and probably around some larger sun. The grandeur of this fragment of truth so overpowered him that he was out of his study, and for some time paced the long street on which his house was situated, regardless of the state of *deshabille* in which he was. From that day his thirst for knowledge increased with each drink he could take at the pure fountain of truth."

Thus it was that long-forgotten volume (Milner's *Tour through Creation*) may be said to have laid the foundation of Dr. Sircar's future eminence as one of the foremost scientific men of his country in the present day.

Dr. Sircar entered the Medical College in 1855, where he remained for 6 years, and became the favourite of all the professors. It was in this wise that he attracted the attention of Dr. Archer, Professor of Ophthalmology: When in his second year, he had to take a relative (a young boy) of his to the out-door dispensary for some eye disease. Dr. Archer was in the habit of testing the knowledge of the students (5th year) who used to attend his clinic, by asking them to answer rather difficult questions on the anatomy and physiology of the eye and on the laws of light. It happened one day that none of the students could answer a question that was put to them about a particular point in the anatomy of the eye. Sircar, who was at a distance taking medicine from the compounder, answered the question in a rather loud voice. "Who is that fellow?" asked Dr. Archer. His students, who knew Sircar, told the Professor that he was a second year student of the College. "A second year student answering my question — call him here". On approaching him, Sircar was literally smothered with various questions about the eye, and the answers being satisfactory, he was asked to attend his clinique every day, though the case for which he had been attending the dispensary had become nearly well.

At the request of the senior students and with the permission of the Professors and the Principal, he delivered a course of lectures on optics, in order to enable the students to better understand the mechanism of the eye as an optical instrument. In this year he delivered a lecture at a meeting of the Bethune Society on the Adaptation of the Human Eye to Distance.

His career in the Medical College was a brilliant one. He obtained medals, prizes and scholarships in Botany, Physiology, Medicine, surgery, and Midwifery. He was sometimes ahead of some of his professors in information in their own specialities. He lost his gold medal in Medical Jurisprudence for having stated in an answer to a question that the lethal dose of arsenic was much larger than stated in books, that men are known who have accustomed themselves to taking it without injury in doses of more than a drachm. This was looked upon by the Professor of Medical Jurisprudence as a gross mistake. The professor evidently had hot read the most recent medical periodical on whose authority Sircar had made the statement.

At the insistence of Dr. Fayrer he went up to the M.D. Examination in 1863, and came out first, the other candidate, the late Dr. Juggobundoo Bose, being second. Dr. Sircar was the second M.D. of the University, the late Dr. Chunder Kumar Dey having been the first.

When Dr. Sircar took to practicing medicine in 1861, he had already been a prominent figure before the public. He had success, so to say, thrust upon him. Among the many distinguished physicians, both European and Indian, in the early sixties, in sagacity and sound judgment, as well as in a thorough acquaintance with all the resources of his art, Dr. Sircar, though still a young man, had few equals and probably no superior. For diseases of the eye he was almost a specialist.

In the same year that Dr. Sircar obtained his M.D. degree, a medical association was established in Calcutta through the exertions of the late Dr. S. G. Chukerbutty, under the name of the Bengal Branch of the British Medical Association. At the opening meeting of this Association, Dr. Sircar in the course of a long and fervent speech, denounced Homoeopathy as one of the systems of quackery. He was elected Secretary of the Association, which office he held for three years, and then elected one of its Vice-Presidents. Dr. Sircar's opinion regarding Homoeopathy changed while he was holding the latter office. On being asked by a friend to review "Morgan's Philosophy of Homoeopathy," for a local lay journal he promised to do it at once! But the perusal of it convinced him that he could and should give no opinion on the book before subjecting homoeopathy to a practical trial. But not knowing it practically himself he could not conscientiously try it. Fortunately at that time Babu Rajendra Dutt, a philanthropic lay Bengali gentleman, who had given him Morgan's pamphlet to read was practicing homoeopathy in Calcutta. Dr. Sircar did not think it *infra dig* to watch cases under this gentleman, and the result was the conviction that homoeopathic medicines, the so-called infinitesimal nothings, did act and act beneficially in removing disease. He thought it his duty to lay this result of his investigation of Homoeopathy before his profession, and to recant what he had said in ignorance of the system at the opening meeting of the Bengal Branch of the British Medical Association. He accordingly read an address in Medicine at its fourth annual meeting, held on the 16th February, 1867, "On the supposed Uncertainty in Medical Science, and on the Relation between Diseases and their Remedial Agents." At the conclusion of this address he said:

"I was so struck with the rapidity and completeness of some of the cures effected by the use of drugs selected after this principle (of similars), that I was compelled, in duty, to watch cases under this peculiar mode of treatment. I became satisfied that the cures were really the effects of the medicines, and not the result of the influence of the imagination, or of a restricted diet, or of the natural progress of the diseases, as I used formerly to believe.

Having been convinced so far, I was induced to make trials of the drugs myself, and for this purpose, I made the peculiar preparations with my own hands, not trusting to the preparations of the shops. I was surprised to find that they do act — and act most marvellously in removing diseased conditions, which yield only tardily to the ordinary mode of treatment.... I do not say that I have succeeded in removing all the diseases that have come under my observation by treatment based on this principle alone. Indeed I must freely admit, that I have failed in numbers of cases, where I was obliged to have recourse to the ordinary treatment, whereby I effected the final cure. The system however, has many recommendations, and I deem it worthy of trial. I feel it, therefore, my duty most humbly to urge upon the profession the necessity of recognizing it as one of our therapeutic systems."

This declaration of faith in Homoeopathy, though so partial, was another great turning-point in the career of Dr. Sircar. He became an outcast in the profession of which he was acknowledgely so conspicuous a member. To the eternal honour, however, of the lay press of India, it must be said that he received its ungrudging and unanimous support. For several months from the day following the fourth annual meeting of the Bengal Branch of the British Medical Association, the man, who had such a large and extensive practice, had not a single call. Some of his best friends, finding that he had ruined his bright prospects, for what they believed was a delusion, became suspicious of his sanity. One of his professors, of whom he was a favourite pupil, admonished him that his bread might be affected. But his calm and firm reply to him and to all else of the sort of low utilitarianism, was — "man must not live by bread alone, but by every word that proceedeth out of the mouth of God."

Seeing that the local and all other professional journals were shut to him, he could find no other way of ventilating his views and of thus convincing his fellowmen of the truth that there is in Homoeopathy than in having a journal of his own. He accordingly started the *Calcutta Journal of Medicine* in January 1868, which he continued to edit to the day of his death. It will be seen that he did not give a sectarian name to the journal which, he announced in the Prospectus, will be conducted on strictly catholic principles, the object being simply and solely the advancement of medical science, though the *Similia Similibus Curantur* law and the infinitesimal posology of Hahnemann will be recognized as the most advanced points yet reached in the domain of therapeutics. The Journal has been the instrument of spreading the cause of Homoeopathy in India. Exchange for the Journal have come mostly unsolicited from England, France, Spain, Germany, Belgium, Italy, Greece, Russia, America, Brazil and Cuba.

The lull in his practice was but temporary. His house began to be more crowded in the mornings than it had ever been before, and his clinic became a regular out-door dispensary in which, for the sake of homoeopathy and the poor, he gave advice and medicines gratis. Owing to the infirmities of age and prostration from frequent attacks of prolonged illness, he was obliged latterly to delegate his duties to his son, Dr. Amrita Lal Sircar, who has been cheerfully devoting for upwards of a dozen years the whole of the mornings to this charitable work, the father occasionally looking after serious cases.

Though by his adoption of homoeoapthy he was plunged in a hot controversy and engaged single-handed in a fierce struggle against a powerful orthodoxy, Dr. Sircar did not forget what he had long been impressed with, that his country could only be regenerated through the cultivation of the sciences. In the opposition to homoeopathy by the old school he saw the grossest ignorance of the highest developments of molecular physics. He was thus stirred by a double incentive to pave the way for scientific research by his countrymen. He accordingly urged them to establish at least one national institution for the purpose, in an article which appeared in this journal for August 1869. The article was so well received both by the native and the European press, that he was encouraged to formulate a scheme of the institution and open subscriptions for the same. The Hindoo Patrist, under the editorship of the late Kristo Dass Pal, gave its powerful and uniform support to the project. It was, however, not till after half a dozen years of incessant begging that he could collect enough money to start the institution in 1876, under the patronage of Lieutenant-Governor, Sir Richard Temple. Dr. Sircar was fortunate from the very beginning in having a true friend in that eminent scientist, Father Lafont of St. Xavier's College. The institution was called the Indian Association for the Cultivation of Science, and the object declared to be the cultivation of science in all its departments, with a view both to its advancement by original research and to its varied applications to the arts and comforts of life.

Had it not been for the generous friendship of Father Lafont the Science Association could not have continue long to exist. The funds collected were just sufficient, with the aid of a house lent by Government, to purchase scientific apparatus for purposes of experimental lectures and to provide for the necessary monthly expenses. They were absolutely inadequate to provide for paid professorships. The Association could only work with honorary lecturers, and Father Laftont and Dr. Sircar were the only men in Calcutta, whose services as such could be confidently counted upon for a number of years. And it reflects no small credit on Father Lafont's love of science and of the natives of this country that he lectured at the Association uninterruptedly for seventeen years, that is, till 1893, after which his numerous avocations and failing health prevented him from continuing his labour of love. He continues, however, to take the liveliest interest in the institution, and is one of its perpetual Vice-Presidents. Dr. Sircar himself could only lecture for three years longer, that is, till 1896, since when, owing to shattered health from an attack of pernicious malarious fever, he was obliged to discontinue most reluctantly the dearest occupation of his life.

The establishment of the Association was hailed by the press, European and native, as an epoch-making event for India. One of the papers (European) had the following in its issue of February 8th, 1877:

"Since Dr. Sircar in 1869 in the "*Calcutta Journal of Medicine* urged the necessity for an institution in this country and under native control for the cultivation of science, up to the present year when his idea has found practical realization, his patient, persistent, and single-minded devotion to the object he had set before him has been such as may well enlist the sympathy and admiration, not only of every devotee of science, but of every friend of human progress, of every admirer of unselfish heroism, of every reformer, and of the every patriot. At one time, his enterprise seemed so hopeless that many men would have set him down, as some we suppose did set him down, as an unpractical dreamer. He seemed like a gifted architect spending his life and genius in planning an edifice for the erection of which no materials existed. Time and the result have already justified him, and we should not doubt that coming generation will preserve his name as one of the worthiest pioneers of the splendid future which we all hope is in store for India. We do not believe that we use the language of exaggeration, but the simplest language to describe a notable fact, when we say that a new era dawned on this country when Dr. Sricar published, and resolved to act upon, his conviction, that "the only method by which the people of India can be essentially improved, by which the human mind can be developed to its full proportions, is by the cultivation of the physical sciences."

The association has made considerable progress since it was started, having got a well-situated local habitation, a good lecture hall, and a well-equipped laboratory. But Dr. Sircar, as its founder, was naturally not satisfied. He was almost in despair of its continued existence so long at least as a few professorships were not endowed. Year after year he appealed for funds, in which he was powerfully supported by successive Lieutenant-Governors and Viceroys, but somehow the appeal seems to have fallen on deaf ears. His countrymen of Bengal, with some honorable exceptions did not appear to realize the magnitude and importance of the Institution, and consequently could not be made to believe that a really large amount of money, much larger than that subscribed, was absolutely necessary to enable the association to fulfill its functions. Referring to the magnificent munificence of Mr. Tata of Bombay for the carrying on of a similar scheme, of which he spoke in terms of glowing sympathy, Dr. Sircar made what he called his final appeal to his countrymen at the twenty-second annual meeting of the Association, held in April, 1899, under the Presidency of Lieutenant Governor of Bengal, as follows:

"It is now for you, my countrymen of Bengal, to determine what you are to do with this Science Association which you have established and which you have advanced so far — whether you are to advance it further or leave it as it is to die of inanition. It cannot contine long without endowed professorships. From the very beginning I have been telling you that in order to enable the Association to do its legitimate work, that of research, you must have men devoting their whole time and attention to special subjects, and that you must provide for them. But somehow or other I have not been able to convince you of this necessity, and the result its that while we are sleeping over a sister presidency has startled the country by what appears to be a new scheme involving an outlay calculated to tax the resources of an empire. Neither the scheme nor the estimate for carrying it out is new. I have been giving out my views of both whenever I could get an opportunity for doing it. I have been giving you accounts of the costs of the various laboratories of the world, of the princely and disinterested gifts for the endowment of new professorships here, or of whole institutes there. But these stories coming from hackneyed lips have apparently had no effect. Now I am feeling that I have come very nearly to the end of my life's journey, I do not see what more I can do than solemnly and imploringly to ask you to take the burden off my shoulders and transfer it to yours".

But apathetic Bengal was unmindful of the preachings of her own prophet. It must be some consolation to Dr. Sircar that though his patriotic endeavours in this matter were disregarded by his own countrymen, they were appreciated by the highest authorities. At the Convocation of the Calcutta University held in 1900, after alluding to Mr Tata's scheme, Lord Curzon, as Chancellor, spoke of Dr. Sircar's institution as follows: "You have, I believe, in your own midst a society, which on a humble scale, because it is only possessed of humble means, attempts to diffuse scientific knowledge among the educated population of Bengal. I allude to the Indian Association for the Cultivation of Science — (applause) — to which Dr. Sircar has, I believe, devoted nearly a quarter of a century of unremitting, and only partially recognized labor (applause). I often wonder why the wealthy patrons of science and culture, with whom Bengal abounds, do not lend a more strenuous helping hand to so worthy and indigenous an institution." At the same convocation, the Vice-Chancellor, Sir Francis Maclean, spoke of Dr. Sircar as "an Indian Votary of Science, upon whom we conferred the honorary degree of Doctor of Law the year before last, (who) has been devoting a lifelong service in preparing the ground for the cultivating of science by his countrymen."

Though he suffered so much from his own profession, Dr. Sircar did not suffer in the least in the estimation of the public or of the Government. His speech at the Education meeting at the Calcutta Town Hall established his reputation as a man of culture, and as an orator of no mean order. "He has been in requisition at every important public meeting" and on each occasion he has displayed the same qualities. "He has been an elected Commissioner of Calcutta for many years and his services on the Municipal Board has always been valuable, especially with his wide knowledge of sanitary science. It was at his motion that a European expert was appointed Health Officer of the city of Calcutta in preference to anative medical officer."

He was appointed a Fellow of the Calcutta University in 1879, and, in recognition of his scholarship and varied attainments, was placed on the Faculty of Arts. He was appointed Sheriff in 1887, the duties of which, with his deputy Babu Ganesh Chunder, he discharged to the entire satisfaction of the Government and the public. By three successive Lieutenant-Governors (Sir Rivers Thompson, Sir Steuart Bailey, Sir Charles Elliott) he was appointed Member of the Bengal Legislative Council from 1887 to 1893.

In 1883 the Government of India, in recognition of his services in the cause of Science, decorated him with the insignia of the Companionship of the Indian Empire (C.I.E.). And in further recognition of the same and other services, in the cause of education generally, the University conferred upon him in 1898 their highest degree, that of Honorary Doctor in the Faculty of Law about which the Chancellor, Lord Elgin, said : "I think that the University has chosen a very appropriate occasion for conferring on Dr. Mahendra Lal Sircar, the Honorary Degree of Doctor of Law in recognition of his eminent services in the cause of Scientific education. Certainly during last year we have been able to observe convulsions of nature on a scale which is almost without parallel. And we know that millions of our fellow-subjects have been suffering from privation from causes of which, we may say, the investigator has yet much to investigate and determine. I congratulate, therefore, the University, as well as Dr. Mahendra Lal Sircar, on the occasion which has been selected for conferring upon him the Honorary Degree of Doctor of Law." The Vice-Chancellor, Mr. Justice Trevelyan, also said: "The degree which has been conferred today upon Dr. Mahendra Lal Sircar was unquestionably his due. The help which he has given to the promotion and better knowledge of science in Bengal by the foundation and maintenance of the Indian Association for the Cultivation of Science itself deserved this recognition. In conferring this degree upon him, we are not merely honoring his labors in the cause of science, we are also endeavouring to repay to some extent the debt which we owe to him. For many years, in spite of the many calls of his professional work, he devoted much of his time to our service. For ten successive years he was a member of our Syndicate, and frequently acted as its President during the absence of the Vice-Chancellor. He was also for four successive years President of the Faculty of Arts."

He was, perhaps, the oldest member of the Asiatic Society of Bengal, was frequently elected a member of its Council, and was its representative on the Board of Trustees of the Indian Museum.

PERSONALITY

A word or two about Dr. Sircar's personal appearance may not be altogether out of place in this sketch, especially regard being had to the fact that he had a remarkable physiognomy. And if human physiognomy has ever been at all anything like an index, good, bad, or indifferent, to the inner man, it must be admitted that Dr. Sircar's outer self was no less striking than his inner self. His Physical which was rather below the middle stature, was gracefully formed; his features had the general expression of simplicity and benevolence, rendered more interesting by a profound philosophic depth and calm which pervaded them. Such eyes, so noble a brow, with its scanty locks so thinly scattered; so symmetrical a profile, so expressive a month, so fine and glowing a complexion; such a combination of manly dignity and beauty, would be hard to match in many another countenance.

It now remains for us to portray the character of this remarkable personality. Perhaps the strongest feature in his character was his sturdy independence, joined to his unflinching devotion to truth and duty. His integrity was most pure, his justice most inflexible;

no motive of interest or consanguinity, of friendship or hatred, could bias his decision. He was a wise, a good, and a great man. His greatness was never shown to greater advantage than in his habitual, outspoken frankness in expressing his views and opinions, which "makes you feel that you are dealing with a man whose character is as transparent as crystal." It was, however, Dr. Sircar's misfortune to be misunderstood by a section of his countrymen. He was believed to have a temper irritable and high-toned. And, admitting he had, did not his reflection and resolution invariably obtain ascendancy over it? Beneath a rough outside, or what was seemingly so to those who did not know him intimately, beat as warm and benevolent a heart as ever beat in a human frame. The tone of harshness which his language as times assumed in conversation ought not to be set down to his unfeeling heart, but to his uncompromising opposition to sham or affectation of any kind; for he had the warmest affections and the kindliest feelings.

In politics Dr. Sircar held advanced views, but he was none of your flaming patriot given to indulging in inane platitudes of India's great past, or in platform blusterings against the powers that be. He never lent his support to Government when in his opinion it was wrong; for as is well-known, on the occasion of the famous Jury meeting, he denounced in no measured terms Sir Charles Elliot's obnoxious notification. Undeterred by the frowns or unseduced by the smiles of Government or the public, he strenuously upheld the cause of truth and justice. In matters of social advancement and reform his views were as pronouncedly liberal, and had their root in his deep and innate regard for woman as the co-equal of man. And that regard found its practical embodiment in the "Rajkumari Leper Asylum." The Asylum was associated with the name of the beloved angel of a wife, but for whose loving administration and tender care "he would have long ceased to be," as he himself said on the occasion of the laying of the foundation-stone of the Asylum by the Lieutenant-Governor, Sir Charles Elliott.

If religion, as Bishop Taylor says, consists not in knowledge, but in a holy life, Dr. Sircar's was pre-eminently a religious life. He never professed a religion in the popular sense of the term. His religion, as appears from his lecture on the "Moral Influence of Physical Science," consisted in an absolute faith in a Supreme Creator and Moral Governor of the Universe, and in the endeavour to live and act with that faith as his pole-star. Thus religion, in its true sense, was ever to him not only his "chief dependence" but his "dearest enjoyment." All through his life he had been an uncompromising opponent of bigotry, intolerance, idolatry, and superstition, and hence it was that he was mistakely looked upon by some of his countrymen as an un-believer in God. Dr. Sircar firmly believed that it was science and science alone which could give man a true conception of God, the foundation of all true religion. In his opinion, "the elevated conception of the Deity, which springs up in the mind from a contemplation of the universe as presented to us by Science, must be incompatible with all unworthy conceptions of Him. In other words, superstition in any shape and a knowledge of physical science cannot exist together." It is noteworthy that Dr. Sircar held Jesus Christ in the highest veneration as the greatest exemplar of Humanity. Dr. Sircar's command over the English language has been no less admired than his high scientific attainments. Whether as a writer or as a speaker he always evinced the most consummate literary predilections. Indeed, every scrap from his pen bears the impress of a skillful literary artist. Dr. Sircar's speeches were greatly admired even by such high personages as Sir Steuart Bayley and Sir John Woodburn. And no wonder, for their rich texture and glowing colours are no less pleasing to the ear than edifying to the soul. A member of the British Parliament, who had heard Dr. Sircar speak, was astonished that one of the best speakers in India was a homoeopath.

The above is an imperfect sketch of the worthy whose life's story would require volumes adequately to unfold. All we have been able to do is to glean stray items of his many-sided life, and to bind them into such sheaves as we could. But still, our labors will not have been in vain, if our young men would endeavour to tread in the footsteps of the heroic and noble soul who, in the words of the poet, had all through life been :

"The tender father and the generous friend;

The pitying heart that feels for human woe;

The dauntless heart that fears no human pride;

The friend of man, to vice alone a foe."

No more graceful or appreciative *critique* on Dr. Sircar's life and genius could be conceived than that penned by a Bengali Bard, whose glowing verse would be a fitting close to our sketch :

"Who risen from the ranks
By wealth of mind ennobled Poverty
Itself: who sowed in gloom and reaped in light;
Successful tiller of the richest fields
Of knowledge; noble builder of the dome
Whence Science spreads her living influence
O'er his fatherland; — kindly heals, — saviour
Of suffering humanity by Art,
Instinct with heavenly mercy, love, and grace"

Nabakrishna Ghose : The Last Day

Dr. Mahendra Lal Sircar, C.I.E., M.D., D. L., was not only the greatest homoeopath of his time in India, but also a great scientist.

He concentrated his life wholly and for ever to the propagation of the principles of homoeopathy. The Calcutta Journal of Medicine edited by him was started in January, 1868 with the ostensible object of disseminating the seeds of homoeopathy in every nook and corner of India. This journal greatly helped homoeopathy to gain a firm footing in the land of his birth.

In the field of physical science, Dr. Sircar has made a great contribution. He may be considered as the pioneer of scientific research in India. Dr. J.C. Bose and Dr. P.C. Ray were also inspired by him.

Recurrent malarial fever and bronchial asthma clouded the evening of his life and he died on February 24, 1904.

Section-S : Dr. Sircar, M.L.

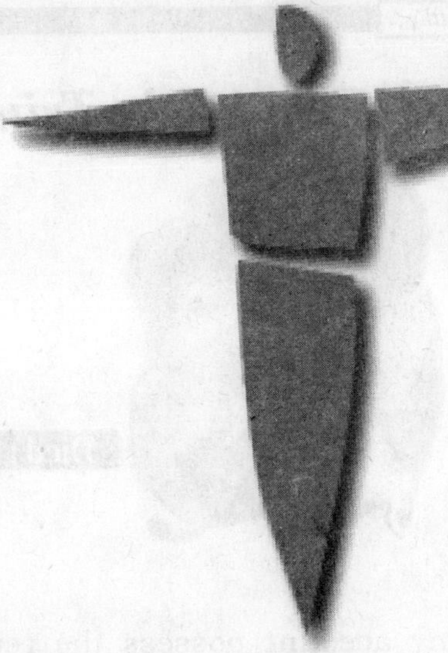

SECTION-T .... Page 257 to 264

T-1 ***Dr. Trinks, Karl Friedrich***
(Born: 08-10-1800 / Died: 05-07-1868) 258

T-2 ***Dr. Tyler, Margaret Lucy***
(Born: 1857 / Died: 21-06-1943) 264

Dr. Karl Friedrich Trinks

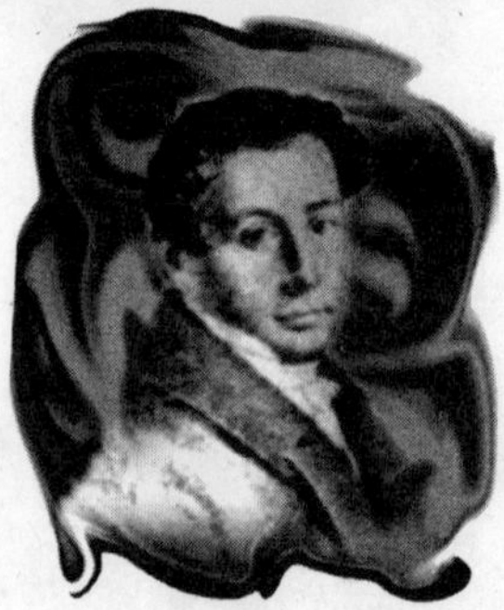

Born : 08-10-1800 Died : 15-07-1868

"I would not on any account possess the reputation of the opponents of Homoeopathy, the reputation on having caused the most ruthless persecutions of their fellow-creatures, because they thought and acted differently from the teachings of Galenic dogmatism."

These were the firm words of K.F. Trinks one of the earliest disciples of Hahnemann and who was among the earliest band of provers, although an earnest lover of homoeopathy he formed the sharpest contrast to Hahnemann in his nature and views, and on certain matters held quite different views from Hahnemann.

The life history of Karl Trinks is the story of poverty and lack of means, contending valiantly and determinedly against seemingly and almost insurmountable obstacles and at last culminating in a glorious triumph like the great Hahnemann, himself.

ANCESTORS & FAMILY

Dr. Karl. F. Trinks was born in a rich family, yet he was never free from wants and economic stress. Daniel Gottfried, his father, was owner of a water-mill. Though his father was a very good person but his mother Marie Rosine was a dominating Lady of miserly and covetous nature. Trinks had only one sister who was four years younger to him.

BIRTH AND CHILDHOOD

Trinks was born on October 8th, 1800. Eythra, a small village, not very far from Leipzig was the birth place of Trinks. When he was 9 years old he was admitted to the village school. He was given primary education by his uncle who later adopted him perceiving

Section-T : Dr. Trinks, Karl Friedrich

that Trinks was a boy of more than ordinary ability and he needed care and help. Under his guidance Trinks learnt Latin, French, History, Mathematics and some branches of natural science. Trinks was very sharp, diligent and meritorious. He learnt Greek language only with the help of a greek grammar book. At this time his uncle placed him in the Grammar School at Merseburg, where he continued his Greek studies under the guidance of one of his school colleagues. In 1814 he attended school at Pastor Hecker in Eythra.

In the school he was loved by all because of his tenacity, earnestness, and attention in the study. His promotion encouraged his uncle very much. But unfortunately his benevolent uncle who cared for all his wants and necessities died of pleuro-pneumonia in 1816. A cloud of bad-fortune came over Trink's head after his uncle's death. With his death his means of living became greatly strained. His mother having always opposed his desire to become a physician in the hope of turning him into a miller restricted his allowances only to six thallers a week which was too pitiably small and was not sufficient for even a part of his most urgent necessities. Therefore, Trinks started earning his livelihood by private tuition and proof reading.

MEDICAL EDUCATION

From childhood Trinks wanted to be a physician. He received some elementary knowledge of practical Surgery and Medicine from a Surgeon of his native village. Trinks helped him in his duties and gathered practical knowledge about medical practice. In 1817 Trinks went to Leipzig and enrolled himself under Dr. Beck, a well-known physician of the time at University at Easter. He studied a lot, made his own extracts and copies. In 1819 he passed his Bachelor's examination with honours. After this he was a favourite student of Prof. Clarus in the Jakob Hospital. Till 1823 he remained at the University and got his M.D. degree on 30th September, 1823.

The title of his thesis was "On some principal obstacles and difficulties in the way of distinguishing and estimating correctly the powers of medicine". The very choice for his thesis paper shows Trinks special interest in Materia Medica, which he considered to be the basis of all medical practice and which he found to be inadequate. Moreover, his thesis paper afforded him opportunity for individual experiments with the separate remedies and for investigations of their dynamic effects.

CONVERSION TO HOMOEOPATHY

Trinks was influenced by homoeopathy through some of Hahnemann's disciples. Although he never attended the great Master's lectures but by 1820 Trinks was friendly with several of Hahnemannian scholars, who were engaged in the proving of drugs like Franz, Homburg and later with Hartmann, Langhammer and others. But amongst all of them Hartlaub had more influence upon the mind of young Trinks with whom he formed a most intimate and enduring friendship. Hartlaub directed him towards the new therapeutic light, and because of his keen critical faculties, he soon realised the advantages of homoeopathy. The influence of the homoeopathic school could be observed by his desire for experiment, for obtaining the specific and dynamic action of drugs. He pointed out the difficulties in the prescription of medicines caused by variations in the susceptibility and power of reaction of the organism, influenced by age, sex, constitution, mode of life and by the combination of drugs in estimating the right nature of medicinal action.

After completing his studies, in 1824 young Trinks went on a tour with his most intimate friend Hartlaub. They visited Dusseldorf, Brussel, Paris then to Germany to Wurzburg and from there to Naumburg where he met Stapf.

MEDICAL PRACTICE

In 1824 Trinks finally settled in Dresden. Trinks and Ernst von Brunnow became known to be the earliest homoeopaths in Dresden. Subsequently Mosdorf, Albrecht, Wofl and Schwarze joined them. It is said that these six homoeopaths started propagating homoeopathic theories in the Saxon capital. After settling at Dresden he went to Bremen for a short time but returned at the end of the same year. His sharp intelligence, deep penetrating knowledge, smartness, wisdom, clear perception and capability as a physician gave him a very prominent position within a very short period of time. The rapidly extended practice of him and his homoeopathic colleagues invited the envy and jealousy of the allopathic physicians; who persecuted him with caricatures and charged him for violating the laws by self-dispensation. He had to face enmity so much so that he was summoned before the magistrate on the charge of dispensing his own medicine.

Inspite of all oppositions Trinks enjoyed a very good practice and a large circle of patients. Throughout the North of Germany

Trinks was regarded as the most distinguished physician who practiced homoeopathy since the time of Hahnemann. He was entrusted with treatment of Princess Caroline of Austria, for which he had to travel to Vienna. Trinks practiced for forty-four years. He had patients from higher classes of society. He was honoured with the title of Medical Councilor. In the year 1863 on July 2nd he received Knightship of the Royal order of Albrecht from the king of Saxony.

Trinks had special affinity and interest in studying two diseases, viz Typhus and Cholera.

MARRIAGE AND FAMILY LIFE

In 1827 this sharp, intellectual fell in love with Auguste Henriette Uhlig, a very beautiful young lady from Merseburg. After a courtship of 3 months, in the company of a few friends at house, and in very simple manner avoiding all ceremonies and outer display, Trinks married her in the month of December. He had a very peaceful domestic life. In 1829 a daughter was born whom he named Elisa. He had great affection for her daughter, and inspite of his heavy engagements he used to devote atleast an hour daily with the little kid. In 1831 his son took birth. Trink's son became a high judicial officer and his daughter got married to a military officer.

TRINKS'S PERSONALITY

The name of Trinks is known and respected by all homoeopaths. His ability and intelligence was admired by the entire homoeopathic world.

He was more a critic than a creative writer. He was a man of practical nature and had a limited interest in art. He had no affection for music or theatre. Even he didn't like poetic literature or the art of painting or sculpture. Neither the joys of companionship nor the holidays could give him recreation. Only books afforded him pleasure and recreation from professional duty that he ever enjoyed.

As a person Trinks was tall and handsome. Earnest expression and deep penetrating look in his blue eyes marked his sharp character. Intellectually he was clear and keen. He was a man of genial disposition and had a good stock of humor which sparkled in his conversation and often appears in writings. He had a very powerful retentive memory. He always preferred the fact than theories, practical than ideal. He loved and practiced homoeopathy because he felt the necessity of development of the principle of pure observation for the practice of medicine. Once he had a very rough discussion with Boenninghausen when he tried mixed medicines into the practice of homoeopathy. He was a supporter of lower dilutions and almost always opposed so-called high potencies. At an early period of the history of homoeopathy when Hahnemann was in the danger of being led away by some of his disciples to promulgate crude and untested notions, Trinks's critical sense prevailed with the founder of Homoeopathy and prevented him committing himself to views that could not stand the test of experience. Trinks opposition did not help him in coming closer to Master Hahnemann. Though, at first, it seemed that he was to join the master more closely but after the publication of Chronic Diseases he criticised Hahnemann acridly.

HIS CONTRIBUTIONS

In 1830 Trinks and the publisher Arnold attended Leipzig Homoeopathic Physicians meeting. This helped to promote the foundation of the Central Association of Homoeopathy. He contributed lot of articles to Hygea and in other homoeopathic journals. Numerous articles appeared from Trink's pen especially in the Homoeopathic Quarterly and the Journal for Homoeopathic Clinics. Trinks contributed a good part of his time in the construction of Homoeopathic Materia Medica.

He edited the *Arzeimittellehre* and *Annalen* with Hartlaub. With Noack he published a Handbook of Materia Medica. Almost regularly he contributed useful articles, practical remarks and criticisms to the homoeopathic periodicals till his death. He was always keen to know latest progress in all branches of medical science.

DEMISE

After the autumn of 1867, this 66 years old physician of dignified and vigorous stature fell sick and at last died on the 15th of July in 1868. He was buried at his native place according to his own desire. On his death, The Dresden Journal (No. 163) wrote:

"In him the Homoeopathic School lost their first reforming authority, and the most important successor of Hahnemann."

TRINKS'S PRINCIPAL WORKS

1824	:	De primaries guibusdam in medica-mentorum viribus recte aestimandis dijudicandisque impediments ac difficultatibus.
1828-1831	:	Materia Medica Pura, 3 volumes.
1829-1830	:	Systematic Representation of the Antipsoric Remedies. In collaboration with C. G. Chr. Hartlaub, 3 volumes.
1830	:	Homoeopathy, An open letter to Hufeland.
1830-1833	:	Annals of the Homoeopathic Clinic, 4 volumes.
1843	:	Hahnemann's Services to Medical Science; (A lecture).
		Manual of Homoeopathic Materia Medica. Volume I (In collaboration with Noack)
1847	:	Manual of Homoeopathic Materia Medica. Volume II & Repertory.
1884	:	Manual of Homoeopathic Materia Medica. Volume III.

Dr. Margaret Lucy Tyler

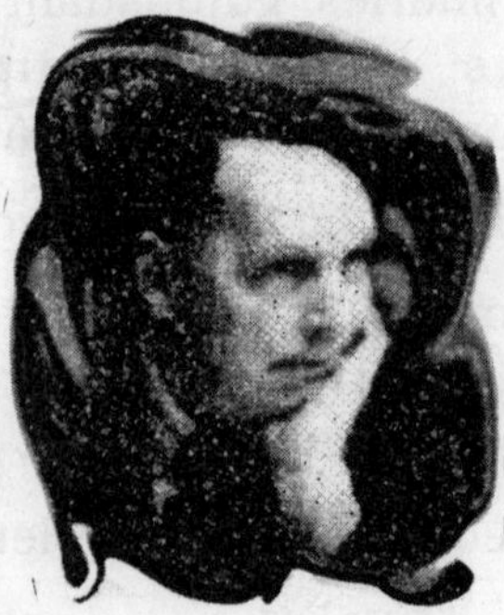

Born : 1857 **Died : 21-06-1943**

Margaret Lucy Tyler was a graduate of both Edinburgh & Brussels universities. She worked at the Royal London Homoeopathic Hospital for forty years. Her speciality was in treating the mentally backward children.

Tyler was a close associate of J.H. Clarke. She used the money, given by her father, Sir Henry Tyler, to fund a Physician's Scholarship to go to Chicago to study with Kent.

She wrote *Homoeopathic Drug Pictures,* which was published in 1942. She also wrote *The Correspondence Course on Homoeopathy.* It was designed for those who could not attend the lectures at the Faculty of Homoeopathy in person.

She died on the 21st of June, 1943 at the age of 86.

SECTION-Y .... Page 265 to 267

Y-1 ***Dr. Yingling, William A.***
(Born: 12-01-1851 / Died: 03-04-1933) 266

Y-2 ***Dr. Younan, W.***
(Born: 1859 / Died: 23-10-1932) 267

Dr. William A. Yingling

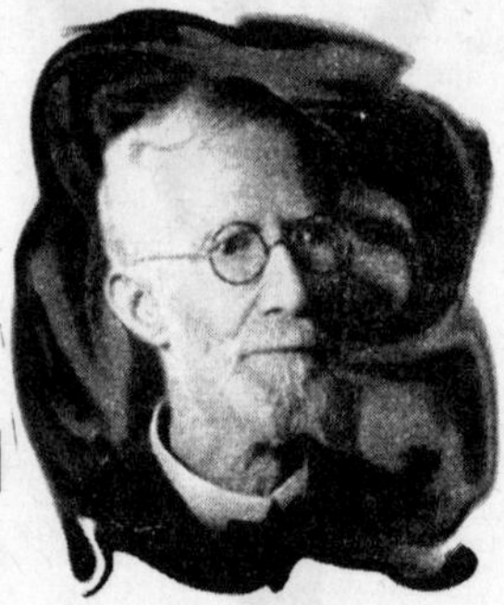

Born : 12-01-1851 **Died : 03-04-1933**

Born on 12th of January, 1851 in Westminster, Maryland, Yingling took his A.B. from Western Maryland College. Because he wanted to become a medical missionary in India, therefore, he took his medical degree at the university of Maryland. Then he studied for the ministry at Northwestern University, Illinois, but due to his ill health he was not able to go to Bombay.

He was minister in Findlay, Ohio for seven years. For the improvement of his ill health he went to Kansas and settled near Dodge City. The town of Nonchalanta, Kansas was named such on his suggestion in 1886. Yingling was involved in the cattle business, but he lost about $75,000 when the Indian Territory was closed to grazing.

He then returned to the practice of medicine to relieve the suffering in the sparsely populated country north of Dodge City. He practiced in Emporia, Kansas and was known as a homoeopathic physician.

He wrote *Accoucheur's Emergency Manual,* which was first published in 1895.

He was sick with paralysis for six months before his death. He died at the age of 82, on 3rd of April, 1933.

Section-Y: Dr. Yingling, William A.

Dr. W. Younan

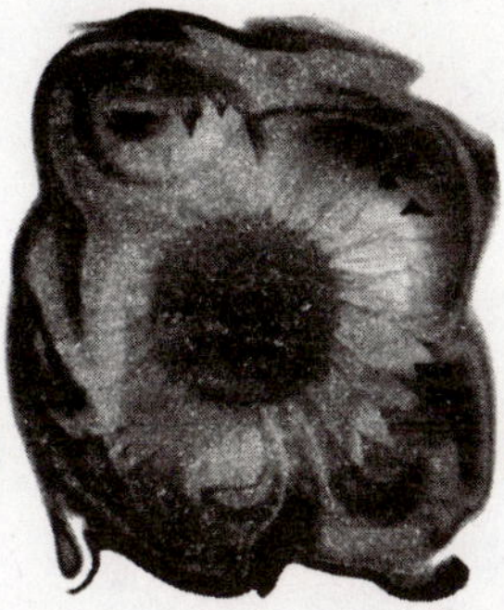

Born : 1859 Died : 23-10-1932

Dr. W. Younan, M.B., C.M. (Edin.), was the son of a police officer in Calcutta, who hailed from Syria. He took his medical degree from Edinburgh University in 1882. He was converted to homoeopathy by the eminent homoeopath, Dr. B.N. Banerjee. He was a master-prescriber who widely popularized homoeopathy, and had thousands of disciples and devotees throughout the Bengal and India. He brought Pandit Motilal Nehru into the folds of homoeopathy by curing his obstinate rhinitis, baffling all other treatments. He never tolerated slightest deviation from Hahnemannian principles. He was the Dean of the Calcutta Homoeopathic Medical College, and President of the Calcutta Homoeopathic Hospital Society and presided over the first All Bengal and Assam Homoeopathic Conference held in Calcutta in 1931. He expired on October 23, 1932, at the ripe age of 73 years.